Living With A Dead Battery

Depression:

A Primer for Family and Professionals

Donald B. Smith

MSSW, DPhil, LCSW (Ret.)

Board Certified Diplomate in Clinical Social Work

GlobalEdAdvance
Press

LIVING WITH A DEAD BATTERY
Depression: A Primer for Family and Professionals

Copyright © 2021 Donald B. Smith

Library of Congress Control Number: 2019941107

Smith, Donald Brian, 1943 -

LIVING WITH A DEAD BATTERY

ISBN 978-1-935434-93-1

Subject Descriptions: 1. Psychology/Psychopathology/Depression 2. Medical/ Psychiatry/Psychopharmacology 3. Self-Help/Mood Disorders/ Depression

Cover design by Global Graphics NYC

Printed in Australia, Brazil, France, Germany, Italy, Poland, Russia, Spain, UK, USA, and wherever there is an Espresso Book Machine

The Press does not have ownership of the contents of a book; this is the author's work and the author owns the copyright. All theory, concepts, constructs, and perspectives are those of the author and not necessarily the Press. They are presented for open and free discussion of the issues involved. All comments and feedback should be directed to the Email: [comments4author@aol.com] and the comments will be forwarded to the author for response.

Order books from www.gea-books.com/bookstore/
or any place good books are sold.

Published by
GlobalEdAdvance Press
a division of
Global Educational Advance, Inc.

Dedication

First, I dedicate this work to my parents, Miller Clayton Smith, Sr. and Claretta (Kay) Brown Smith, who, although not always understanding my depression, stood with me in my years of struggle with support and caring love.

Second, I dedicate this work to the psychiatrists with whom I worked over the 40 plus years in the field of mental health care and treatment: Colonel Ted Cook, MD of Brooke Army Medical Center, Texas; Robert Callaway, MD, Marion Young, MD of Joseph W. Johnson Community Mental Health Center, Robert Spaulding, MD, D. Ross Campbell, MD, Jim Varner, MD; William Greer, MD of Valley Psychiatric Hospital, all of Chattanooga, Tennessee; Frank Kulik, MD and Wolf Glaser, MD, Loyd Noland Hospital, Birmingham, Alabama. These excellent psychiatrists were beneficial to me in learning about or expanding my knowledge of mental illness and more importantly of mental health. Through them, what competence as a clinical social worker I may have attained was learned, honed and refined. I owe my clinical career to these psychiatrists.

Table of Contents

Foreword

A Useful Tool

This is a work that is well written, professionally presented and scientifically accurate. It is a pleasure to read and will prove to be of singular assistance to those who are engaged in helping those who are afflicted with the foul darkness of depression.

The work is up to date on the most recent methods and instruments of professional intervention in this ubiquitous disorder. It is a disorder that will fill a majority of the schedules of those in consulting offices or pastoral studies. It will become a necessary compendium for every therapist and pastor who engages in a counselling ministry. Such practitioners will see cases of depression, in a plethora of forms and disguises – psychological, somatic and spiritual – and in all probability such cases will constitute the majority of those who come seeking help and relief.

This author is obviously knowledgeable of the purely medical and psychological elements of depression. The author in a very skillful and professional way and one that reflects years of clinical experience refutes the lie which unfortunately is common among Evangelicals that all depression is a symptom of a spiritual problem and must be dealt with by spiritual or pseudo-spiritual means. This is a view that causes much harm and aggravation of the clinical phenomenology among many pastors and poorly educated would-be psychotherapists and counsellors today.

I have seen too many examples of patients suffering from depression, which was the result of purely psychological or physical causes, devastated by accusation and opinions that the disorder constituted evidence that there must be sin in the life of the suffering individual. Such unfortunate individuals are then exhorted to go and confess their sin and the depression will be cured. Often there is nothing to confess and as result the individual feels abandoned by both God and man and becomes convinced that there is no available forgiveness. This eventuates in aggravation and deepening of the depressed state. We can be thankful that this author will not fall into this faux pas and has demonstrated that he has a forged clinical acumen.

The author's detailed review of the whole subject of depression is extremely useful. He explicates the different types of depression, as well as the various methods of intervention available, both psychological and medical. Accurate Differential Diagnosis is the prerequisite to any form of therapy. In this connection it would have been useful if the author had included information on the spiritual roots of some forms of depression since this is one of the commonest areas in which there is mis-diagnosis and mis-directed intervention.

I am more than impressed with the author's knowledge of the recent advances in psychiatric intervention, especially in the area of current medications. The intricacies of neuro-chemistry is a difficult field and this author has done a remarkable service for the busy pastor and therapist in rendering the area of modern chemical intervention in the form of anti-depressants and tranquilizers more easily understood and therefore more available.

This book is one I can recommend without any reservation as an *'on-the-desk'* compendium for every psychotherapist, counsellor, psychologist and psychiatrist, especially those who are students or entering the field. Here they will find a source of information that is immediately available, accurate, useful and invaluable. Even those who have experience in the field will find the succinct review of the neuro-chemical agents valuable. The author has done us a service by his intense review of the current literature and the indications for the use of medications and other methods of intervention currently available.

One of the most useful volumes for the practicing therapist that I have seen for a long time!

— **E. Basil Jackson, MD, ThD, PhD, JD**
Psychiatry & Neurology - Psychiatry

You know, I've seen a lot of people distancing themselves from people dealing with depression; well, that's not okay. By turning your back, you'll only complicate things and motivate the thought "I don't matter. People hate, its better if I just leave earth" to that depressed person. Oh well, just in case you don't know, depression isn't contagious. It's pretty much not a disease, it's just a mental illness that comes and goes. All you have to do is stay strong and try to stay positive. Don't let depression take control over your life, you are the only who's in control over your life. Don't let depression win.

-Kim Taehyung
BTS, Big Hit Entertainment
Seoul, Korea

BTS's RM and Suga talk mental health, depression, and connecting with fans

Leah Greenblatt

March 29, 2019 at 03:00 PM EDT

https://ew.com/music/2019/03/29/bts-rm-suga-mental-health/

Pop stardom may be a dream job, but the artists who make it still struggle with many of the same realities their fans do.

This week's EW cover stars BTS have made a point of bringing the feelings nearly everyone experiences at some point in their lives — sadness, loneliness, low self-esteem — into the light, both in their song lyrics and in the missions they support, like their Love Myself campaign (which they presented at a United Nations youth summit last September) and violence partnership with UNICEF.

During a recent interview at the Seoul headquarters of their record label Big Hit Entertainment, the band sat down with EW to cover a whole range of topics (their experience at the Grammys, their secret hobbies, why they love John Cena). But they got serious, too, on the topic of mental health.

Asked whether they found it harder or easier as celebrities to put their private pain out there in songs and on social media, Suga was adamant: *"We feel that people who have the platform to talk about those things really should talk more, because they say depression is something where you go to the hospital and you're diagnosed, but you can't really know until the doctor talks to you.*

"So I think for not just us but other celebrities," he goes on, *"if they talk about it openly — if they talk about depression for example like it's the common cold, then it becomes more*

and more accepted if it's a common disorder like the cold. More and more, I think artists or celebrities who have a voice should talk about these problems and bring it up to the surface.

RM elaborates: *"That's why we have the concept Love Yourself. We don't want to preach 'Do this or don't do that,' because that's not the way that we want to spread our message. Like for example, say, Anna from New York or Marc from Rio or me or you, we have different looks, different races, different parents and backgrounds, different weather, whatever. Everything's different."*

"We're born with different lives," he continues, *"but you cannot choose some things. So we thought that love, the real meaning of it, starts with loving ourselves and accepting some ironies and some destinies that we have from the very start. But we never chose that, so instead of preaching or [giving] orders, that's why we committed to loving yourself and that's why I started with 'I'm just an ordinary boy from city near Seoul in South Korea' at our U.N. speech."*

For the band, the music is the message, too — and it goes both ways: *"Our greatest influence,"* says Suga, *"and where we draw our strength and our comfort and our joy is the fans, So we always have that in mind when we make our music, and I think our fans are also able to get that same strength or joy."*

For more on BTS, *pick up the new issue of* Entertainment Weekly *on stands Friday, buy it now, or scoop up our limited-edition* BTS *poster. And don't forget to subscribe for more exclusive interviews and photos, only in* EW.

Introduction

Depression: A Primer for Families and Professionals

The first thing that a seeker or student of mental health should know is this: Depression is real, complicated, and greatly misunderstood. Depression is painful. People many times fail to recognize the complex of symptoms that creates a state of depression. The depressive's family, friends, employers and co-workers, associates in social and civic arenas and religious organizations, and frequently even the depressed person often misunderstand depression.

Because of these facts, a significant amount of disharmony, hurt, and anger may result. Lack of support of many kinds goes lacking. Criticism and unmet expectations create difficulty in relationships. Depression can make everyone involved in it unhappy and miserable.

This raises the question about what depression is, how to recognize it, what are the causes, and what actions to take regarding it. As previously stated, depression is complicated with accompanying spheres of physical, biological, chemical, mental, emotional, social, and psychological dynamics. To gain understanding of depression requires one to understand how these dynamics play out in daily lives.

For the person affected by depression and for those interacting with the depressed person, both good news and bad news exists. First, the good news: Treatment for depression may bring and maintain a satisfactory life. Now, the bad news: In some instances of severe depression, the condition may never be resolved. Therapeutic interventions may be a life-long requirement.

This book provides both nonprofessional and professional readers a clear, consistent, concise, and correct presentation of depression by one who has a lifetime of personal experience and a professional career of care, treatment, and support for people with depression and their family and friends. The book provides foundational concepts about depression and offers the reader the opportunity to gain insight into the behaviors and dynamics resulting from this insidious condition.

Many people believe they understand depression. Some do. Most do not. Although great gains have occurred over the past 50 years in understanding and treating depression, the condition remains as a prominent mental health issue worldwide. Depression affects family life, community efforts at resolving a number of local issues, and policy decisions in the arenas of public health, mental health, economics, social welfare, and politics.

Two commonly distinct forms of depression exist— persistent depressive disorder (once known as common depression and dysthymia) and Major Depressive Disorder (major depression). Both can be devastating conditions if left unresolved or untreated. One form or the other for many people becomes that life-long struggle previously mentioned. Both are similar except for that one condition—longevity and severity.

Causal factors for depression may be four-fold. One, two, or all four factors may be at play in the condition. For this reason, the condition requires a comprehensive clinical, social, and medical evaluation to determine treatment, care, and support options. These four causal factors are physical trauma, biological change, emotional upset and genetic make up.

For most of us, we think that some type of mental or emotional breakdown is the cause of depression. Few of us know that a physical trauma—a broken bone, or a hormonal shift may cause a state of depression in an individual. The repercussions of this circumstance can be staggering and costly in medical costs and family discord, simply because depression was not or was too late recognized.

Science has come a long way in the idea of genetic predisposition of some individuals toward depression. We have long known that in many instances a familial predisposition tended toward depression in some family members. In the past, we have considered family tendencies toward depression were more environmental and emotional conditions.

However, recent research has found certain genetic defects seem to be causal to depression and other more severe disorders such as schizophrenia. This break-through in science allows a greater understanding of why some people do not fully respond to various treatment interventions and do not totally recover from a major depressive episode. We seem to have far to go.

As the reader, one should approach this study with openness and inquiry. Do not expect to become an expert in the diagnosis and treatment of depression. However, consider this as the first step in gaining insight into the condition, its manifestation, and its dynamic.

REVIEW QUESTIONS

(written or discussion)

1. What is the first thing one should know about depression?

2. What are some results of depression as it occurs in interpersonal relationships?

3. Name the spheres mentioned in the text in which the dynamic of depression may be at work.

4. Can you think of any others spheres in which depression may affect quality of life?

5. Is depression treatable?

6. Is depression curable?

7. What are the types of depression?

8. What are the 4 essential causes for depression?

CLASS DISCUSSION

What do you consider as symptoms of depression? Someone in the class should serve as recorder, to compose and keep a list for further discussion in a later class. Keep the list available.

1

What Is Depression?

Depression is a common and serious medical illness that negatively affects how one feels, the way one thinks and how one acts. Depression takes on many forms. Fortunately, it is also treatable.

Depression causes feelings of sadness and/or a loss of interest in activities once enjoyed. It can lead to a variety of emotional and physical problems and can decrease a person's ability to function at work and at home. Depression is more than just a "blue Monday," or feeling sad or down for a day or two. That is not depression. At the extreme end of the spectrum, suicide can result.

Depression is a very debilitating disorder that affects a large number of people worldwide. Depression can cause someone to feel utterly dispirited or dejected. Depression is a state of cast down, disheartened, demoralized, crushed, desolate, or oppressed.

Depression may cause thoughts and feelings of pushed down or pulled down into a lowered state of existence. Depression may actually paralyze a person's cognitive and emotional functioning. It can drain one physically of energy and mobility.

According to the United States National Institute of Mental Health (NIMH), depression is one of the most common mental disorders in the United States.[1] "An estimated 16.2 million adults in the United States had at least one major depressive episode. This number represented 6.7% of all U.S. adults," according to NIMH.[2]

Current research suggests that a combination of genetic, biological, environmental, and psychological factors causes depression.[3] We will take a nonprofessional's view of these causal factors.

The World Health Organization has characterized depression as one of the most disabling disorders in the world, affecting roughly one in five women and one in ten men at some point in their lifetime. Estimates suggest that 21% of women and 12% of men in the United States experience an episode of depression at some point in their lifetime.

Depression can happen at any age, but often begins in late adolescence or early adulthood. We now recognize depression as occurring in children and early adolescents, although it sometimes presents with more prominent irritability than low mood.

The NIMH website states "An estimated 3.1 million adolescents aged 12 to 17 in the United States had at least one major depressive episode. This number represented 12.8% of the U.S. population aged 12 to 17. The prevalence of major depressive episode was higher among adolescent females (19.4%) compared to males (6.4%). The prevalence of major depressive episode was

1   https://www.nimh.nih.gov/health/topics/depression/index
2   https://www.nimh.nih.gov/health/statistics/major-depression
3   http://www.mentalhealthamerica.net/conditions/depression

highest among adolescents reporting two or more races (13.8%)."[4]

Many chronic mood and anxiety disorders in adults begin as high levels of anxiety in children. With children, a characteristic symptom is pain in the stomach.

Depression in midlife or older adults can occur with other serious medical illnesses, such as diabetes, cancer, heart disease, and Parkinson's disease. These conditions are often worse when depression is present. Sometimes medications taken for these physical illnesses may cause side effects that contribute to depression. Depression may also appear like symptoms of dementia and Alzheimer's disease and must be considered and ruled out by the diagnosing physician prior to a diagnosis of dementia or Alzheimer's.

Depression, then, presents itself as a physical or mental disorder. Depression is commonly a chemical imbalance in the brain that affects one's ability to move, to use cognitive functions, or to view positively the world as a whole.

DOMAINS OF DEVELOPMENT AND FUNCTION

A Biblical Proverb states that as a person thinks, so is he. Put another way, our thinking controls who and what we are. This statement has important ramifications in treating some forms of persistent depressive disorder, especially without the use of medications, as many psychologists prefer.

Consider that people develop and function in what we call three domains—the Affective Domain, the

4   https://www.nimh.nih.gov/health/statistics/major-depression. shtml

Behavioral Domain, and the Cognitive Domain. These domains represent the way individuals feel, behave, and think. What are the primary traits or characteristics of these three domains?

The Affective Domain is the domain of moods, attitudes, and emotions. This domain reflects these traits primarily in one's affect—or the expressions and body postures. Affect is emotion or desire, especially as influencing behavior or action.

"One is affectionate." "He has a flat affect—showing no animation or emotion." "The music visibly affected her."

The Behavioral Domain centers in the behaviors one presents. We consider behaviors as appropriate or inappropriate. They can be helpful, not helpful, or self-defeating. One's emotions strongly and primarily control behaviors. Emotional needs take priority over reasoning.

The Cognitive Domain is the domain of the mind. Thinking, reasoning, deciding, choosing, and organizing are cognitive processes. The battle with depression is largely the battle for cognition.

These, then, are the ABC's of the self. Affective is feeling, Behavioral is doing, and Cognitive is thinking. The effects of these three domains on the self extend into all areas of human development and function.

WHERE DIAGNOSES COME FROM

The *Diagnostic and Statistical Manual* of Mental Disorders (DSM) is the handbook used by health care professionals in the United States and much of the world as the authoritative guide to the *diagnosis* of mental disorders. DSM contains descriptions, symptoms, and other criteria for diagnosing mental disorders. The American Psychiatric Association publishes it. Currently the DSM is in its fifth edition and known commonly as the DSM-5.

SUMMARY

Depression is a common, misunderstood, and treatable disorder that affects mood, feelings, behavior, and thinking. Depression can make an individual dysfunctional in many areas of life. Depression may appear as early as childhood and late as onset of retirement.

Depression affects three domains of development and function. Depression influences affective, behavioral, and cognitive functioning. As a result, depression can present itself as either a physical, behavioral, thinking, or mood disruption. Depression takes many forms.

REVIEW QUESTIONS

(written or discussion)

1. Name and describe three domains of human development and function.

2. Match the following:

   a. Affect   i. Thinking
   b. Behavior   ii. Feeling
   c. Cognition   iii. Doing

3. In what ways can depression manifest in an individual?

4. T F Depression is a common disorder that is simple and easily understood.

5. T F More than one form of depression exists?

6. T F One who has been sad or blue for a couple of days because of a problem or loss should be considered depressed.

7. T F A child cannot experience depression because the child has not had significant life experience in which depression is rooted.

CLASS DISCUSSION

What do you know about depression? Do you know someone who has depression?

Anger or Rage	Impaired Memory or Recall
Anxiety	Insomnia
Chronic Pain	Irritability
Crying for no Apparent Reason	Labile Mood (mood swings)
Decreased/Increased Appetite	Lack of Energy
Decreased/Increased Sleep	Listlessness (may seem lazy)
Decreased/Increased Weight	Loneliness even around people
Fatalism	Loss of interest in sexual activity
Feeling Totally Discouraged	Loss of muscle tone for standing
Feeling Overwhelmed	Lost Interest in favorite activity
Feelings of Helplessness	Moodiness
Feelings of Hopelessness	Negativity
Feelings of Uselessness	Periods of short or rapid breath
Gastrointestinal Problems	Sadness – no apparent reason
Hostility	Sense of Despair
Hypochondria	Social isolation
Impaired Concentration	Suicidal Ideas or Thoughts
Impaired Thinking	Withdrawal
Impaired Decision-making	World better off without me

Figure 1: Characteristic Symptoms of Depression

2

Symptoms Of Depression

The symptoms of depression are many. Not everyone has all these symptoms. Some do. Not everyone experiencing some of these symptoms have a form of depression. My friend Jim said, "We all feel that way sometimes." That, of course, may be a true statement.

We all go through periods of sadness, of sleeplessness, of lack of energy, and of discouragement. Those are all part of the range of human emotions that human beings experience. Frustration with the depressed person or in the depressed person oneself may come out in outbursts of anger. The difference between these individuals as representative of "all of us" and those of us who are depressed in some clinically diagnosed form is significant. The difference is the length of time a depressed person consistently and continuously experiences these symptoms in comparison to "us all."

Consider depression as a syndrome—a disorder having a set of symptoms. A combination of these symptoms increases the likelihood of depression. Seldom does having one or two interrelated symptoms lead to a diagnosis of depression. This fact is another key to understanding depressive states.

Figure 1 shows a near exhaustive list of symptoms that in combination may indicate the presence of some form of depression. Remember, a combination of symptoms extended for up to 2 weeks or longer, and not one or two symptoms from time to time, indicates the occurrence of depression. Get to know this list of 36 symptoms.

DESCRIBING THE SYMPTOMATIC BEHAVIORS

Although we generally know what certain words mean, sometimes they take on a more specific or even different understanding or meaning in a medical setting. For example, we generally think of something being positive as a good thing. However, in medicine a positive reading of a test—meaning the patient has the condition, is not good.

Acute is another example. In lay terms, acute means sharp or intense. In a clinical setting acute means something entirely. It means of recent onset and of short endurance versus chronic, meaning long-standing or long existing.

Having a clearer understanding of how these words or conditions are used helps in deciding courses of action. Find a complete list of terms found in this book in the Word List (Appendix 1).

We all become angry at times. When the anger is explosive, dangerous, or long-standing, especially for no apparent reason, this anger or even rage, may be symptomatic of depression or some other mental health issue. Some form of intervention seems likely.

We commonly think of anxiety as "a feeling of worry, nervousness, or unease, typically about an imminent event or something with an uncertain outcome." In clinical terms, though, anxiety is "a nervous disorder characterized by a state of excessive uneasiness and apprehension, typically with compulsive behavior or panic attacks." The feelings of anxiety and of fear may be the same feelings but with fear, one knows the cause of the feeling and in anxiety, the cause may be unknown.

Sometimes people complain of ongoing pain in their stomach, back or other body part. A specific cause cannot be determined for this chronic pain. We often think these people are faking it or say, "It's all in her head."

Often we call this person a hypochondriac. Alternatively, he just wants attention. They are making it up.

For many people with unexplained on-going pain, the pain is real. It is not just in the head or "made up." Depression can cause this pain not related to physical illness, muscle strain, fractures, or injury.

Sometimes one cries for no apparent reason. "Why are you crying? What's wrong?" "It's nothing." "I don't know." "There must be something."

Ever had that conversation with someone? Chances are that other person was depressed. Crying for no apparent reason can be symptomatic of depression. In addition, sadness for no apparent reason can be a symptom of depression.

Changes in appetite, weight (without dieting), and sleep patterns are very good indicators that something is going on in a person's life. Sometimes people seek comfort from their sorrows by eating. Over an extended time, this behavior may indicate depression or an eating disorder.

Depression can affect the functions of the brain. These include problems with memory, recall, concentration, and decision-making. Thinking sometimes gets jumbled.

Irritability, hostility, negativity, moodiness, and mood swings commonly occur in people with depression. These traits are strong indicators of depression. One with depression cannot just think or be positive.

Problems with stomach or intestines may be a direct result of depression. According to psychiatrist, the late D. Ross Campbell, MD[5], of Chattanooga, Tennessee, a sure symptom of depression in adolescents is a pain just below the sternum, in the stomach. Gastritis, incontinence and other stomach and bowel problems may reflect the potential for a diagnosis of depression.

Of course, other causes may exist for these conditions. A physician can make those determinations. That is why it is important to report everything going on, regardless of whether the individual or family member thinks it important.

When a person no longer takes an interest in his favorite pastimes or her favorite social activities, or when going out with the guys or girls becomes a burden, depression might be suspected. Loss of interest in hobbies, events, and friendship activities, even church attendance, all suggest depression might exist in the

---

5   Campbell, D. Ross, MD in patient case conference, Valley Psychiatric Hospital, Chattanooga TN, 1979

individual. Social withdrawal and isolation frequently result from depression.

When an individual neglects personal hygiene for significant periods, one can suspect depression. Loss of interest in one's appearance, lack of shaving, lack of bathing or showering, not doing one's nails or hair all may indicate a person is experiencing a form of depression.

Remember, most people may experience one or more of these symptoms from time to time. Such an occurrence for a few days may not be significant. However, when one experiences these symptoms over weeks, when these symptoms affect one's daily living skills and activities, depression in some form may be indicated.

REPORTING SYMPTOMATIC BEHAVIORS

To repeat for emphasis, we all can have one or more of these symptoms during the course of our lives. Having one or two of these symptoms from time to time does not indicate depression. Persistent occurrence or reoccurrence of several of these symptoms may be indicative of clinical depression (persistent depressive disorder or recurrent major depression.)

Often some of these symptoms are viewed as a bad attitude, an indifference, or just not trying. Many times these symptoms are not reported to clinicians. That is the reason a full description of the individual is necessary—in appearance, in behavior, and in conversation.

The social worker's exhaustive Social History has a significant role to play in describing the new client or patient. The social history delves into all aspects of the depressed person's life—the thoughts, the feelings, and the behavior, in a structured and comprehensive manner.

A checklist provides one way for a person to determine whether to consult with a physician about depression. This checklist is from the Zung Self-Rating Depression Scale[6] (See Appendix 2). These are some considerations regarding seeing a licensed health care professional for an actual evaluation for depression. This self-rating scale provides only a rule of thumb check.

Licensed health care professions may provide the complete rating scale and other screening and assessment tools. The health care professional uses this tool and provides supervision for a patient who self-administers this test. People self-administering this test need consultation with a health care professional.

A qualified licensed health care professional such as a psychiatrist, physician, psychologist, psychiatric registered nurse, or licensed clinical social worker makes a proper evaluation for depression. When seeking help for screening for depression, inform the clinician of the symptoms only. Do not attempt to self-diagnose or suggest to the clinician what may be going on.

By stating only the symptomatic behaviors listed above, the reporter provides the evaluator the information necessary to rule out other conditions that may confuse the evaluation process. Family accompanying someone suspected of experiencing depression should allow that person to respond in her or his own way. Resist the urge

6   Zung, W. W. K., MD, Arch Gen Psychiatry, 1965, 12 (1), 63-70

to prompt or correct the respondent or to explain her or his responses. The evaluator uses the responses to evaluate for other conditions and the degree or level of impairment.

Remember, there are no "correct" answers for the evaluation. The nature and the accuracy of the response is part of the evaluation process.

SUMMARY

The list of characteristics symptoms of depression is a long one. Frequently some of these symptoms may not be associated with depressive disorders. That is one reason an assessment or a diagnosis of depression is missed.

All too often, we consider someone as lazy, indifferent, sullen, or moody. They seem lazy and irresponsible. The have a bad attitude.

Symptoms of depression may be physical, mental, social or emotional in nature. Depressive disorders are not only mental or emotional conditions. Serious biochemical or physical situations may cause by depression.

REVIEW QUESTIONS

(written or discussion)

1. Name 10 characteristic symptoms of depression.

2. T F One or two symptoms of depression experienced over a period of 3 to 4 days means a person is depressed.

3. T F One should report unrelated or insignificant behaviors to the clinician even though the individual thinks them unimportant.

4. T F We all go through periods of sadness, of sleeplessness, of lack of energy, of discouragement.

5. When should we suspect that a person has depression rather than just having a bad time?

CLASS DISCUSSION

Pull out your list of symptoms of depression you compiled as a group in Chapter 1. How does your list compare with what was presented in this Chapter? What new insights have you gained? In what areas do you need more information?

3

How Depression Works

Now that we have identified the symptoms of depression, the question arises about how depression causes these symptoms. In other words, how does depression work? This chapter deals with this question.

THE EXAMPLE OF THE AUTOMOBILE

To begin, let us look at the operation of an automobile. We will then draw an analogy. This approach should help explain how depression works in one's body.

An automobile has a number of operating systems. They include a fuel system, a transmission system, a braking system, a cooling system and an electrical system, among others. In working together and in coordination, the auto functions properly and well.

For our example, we will look at part of the electrical system. That system includes such things as the battery, the starter, the alternator, the voltage regulator, the radio/tape deck/DVD player, and the lights. Let us look at each component.

First, consider the battery. The battery is the energy storage unit. Electrical energy is stored in the battery. The interaction of sulfuric acid and lead plates creates energy internal to the battery. A fully charged battery is necessary for proper operation of the vehicle.

Next, think about the starter. The starter is the element that causes the capacity for movement in the vehicle. With a faulty starter, the motor does not engage and operation (movement) of the automobile does not happen.

Once the motor is engaged and operating, the alternator sends energy back into the battery. This process recharges the battery. If the alternator is defective, the battery must utilize only the energy that is contained within it and eventually runs down.

After the starter has started the motor and the alternator is returning electrical current back into the battery, other units within the electrical system function properly. These include the radio and the tape deck or DVD player, the headlights, taillights, and dashboard lights, the windshield wipers and the fan for heating or cooling. With a discharged battery, these functions do not happen.

The other accessories are dependent upon the flow of current. With insufficient flow of energy, they do not operate properly or even at all. For this example, we will consider only the headlights and the tape deck or DVD player.

As a mechanic at one point in his life, the author operated a full service auto service and fueling station. Often he received calls regarding a customer having "a dead battery." The car would not start.

As a note, this call and report compares to a patient or family member telling the physician what he or she thinks is wrong. The suggestion may be "misdiagnosis." The mechanic must make the diagnosis.

A diagnostic process was necessary to determine exactly what was wrong. The author could have "taken the customer's word" that the problem was a dead battery and merely replaced the battery. If the old battery were still good, its costly replacement would have fixed nothing, but the author would have made money off the customer.

However, a diagnostic procedure would reveal the actual cause of the problem—why the automobile was not operating, as it should. In the case of a dead battery, a simple test could rule out several problems. Ruling out a condition is part of the diagnostic process.

In the case of the automobile not starting, the test requires a simple procedure. Turn on the headlights. Turn the key to start the car. What happens?

If the battery is discharged (or dead), all the energy that might remain in the battery (residual energy) is directed toward the starter. If that is the case, sufficient electricity to energize the headlights does not exist. That means a discharged battery.

However, if when activating the starter, the headlights do not dim out, sufficient electrical current is available to operate the lights, DVD player, and other functions in the car. The problem for the car not starting is not the battery but the starter.

One might call this process a differential diagnosis. One looks at different symptoms and potential problems to determine what is problematic with the vehicle. Of course, if the battery has discharged, further testing may be required to determine the cause.

The cause of the discharge in the battery might be due to a faulty alternator or voltage regulator. It might mean the battery acid spent out and needs re-supply. Alternatively, it might mean the battery has a dead cell, meaning a dead battery.

Figure 2 shows a diagram of what we have just described in terms of the automotive electrical system.

Electrical System of a Modern Automobile

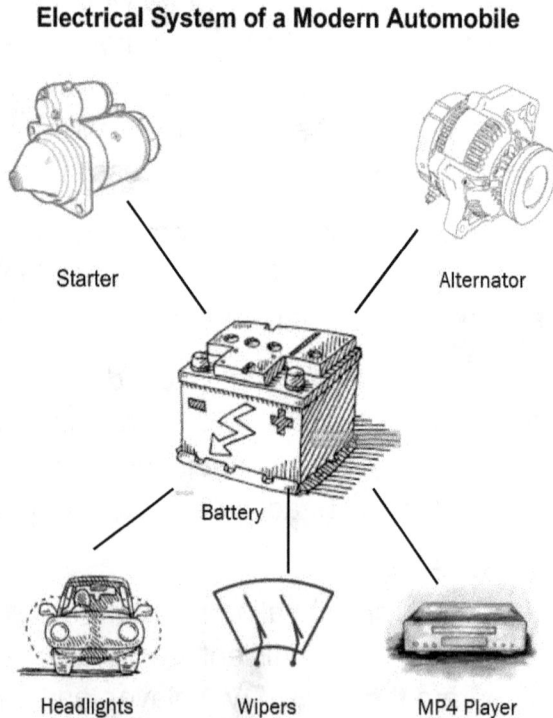

Starter   Alternator

Battery

Headlights   Wipers   MP4 Player

Figure 2: Automobile Electrical Systems

The battery is the source of energy. The starter initiates movement. The alternator recharges the electrical system and battery. The tape deck or the DVD plays back whatever has been impressed upon it. The headlights allow us to see and to find our way in the darkness.

NEUROTRANSMITTERS AND SYNAPSES

At this point, a definition seems in order. The word is neurotransmitters. Neurotransmitters are crucial for the transmission of energy impulses along a nerve in the brain.

A neurotransmitter is a chemical substance released at the end of a nerve fiber by the arrival of a nerve impulse and, by diffusing across the synapse or junction, causes the transfer of the impulse to another nerve fiber, a muscle fiber, or some other structure. It transmits signals across a chemical synapse, such as a neuromuscular junction, from one neuron (nerve cell) to another "target" neuron, muscle cell, or gland cell. Synaptic vesicles in synapses release neurotransmitters into the synaptic cleft and received by receptors on the target cells.

Though the brain has billions of nerve cells, they do not actually touch – thus the job of neurotransmitters to bring messages back and forth. Because neurotransmitters can affect a specific area of the brain, including thinking, behavior or mood, their malfunctions can cause effects ranging from mood swings to aggression and anxiety. Many neurotransmitters exist in the brain, but those most studied in relation to mental disorders are dopamine, acetylcholine, Gamma-amino butyric acid (GABA), noradrenalin (norepinephrine) and serotonin.

HOW DEPRESSION WORKS IN THE BODY

Now we turn to depression and the individual's function. Substitute the brain for the battery, the starter for physical movement, neurotransmitters, and that tape or DVD player for memory. We could even substitute windshield wipers for clear vision of the surroundings and situation. The example is simplistic but helps visualize what is transpiring in depressive episodes.

When a person has depression, the brain energy level may deplete. Sometimes this reduced brain energy can occur in daily living situations but with rest and adequate diet, one recovers after a day or two. Our body makes a temporary adjustment.

However, with depression we are looking at a discharged battery not recharging. The energy level depletes. One does not have the energy for the body to function properly.

The brain is the source of thought and movement. It needs an adequate supply of energy to operate its systems. Low energy or insufficient energy we will call, in our example, depression.

With depression, most of what little energy that exists is directed to physical movement, physical activity. That means the "starter" is consuming what electrical impulses the brain is sending out. That is why lack of energy can be a strong indicator of depression when other symptoms are involved.

Because of insufficient energy, one may not be able to exercise, to work, or even to get out of bed. This individual is not lazy. Telling this person just to "make yourself do it" is not at all helpful and shows clear misunderstanding of depression.

Also because of insufficient energy and the fact that existing energy is directed toward physical movement, the individual's ability to see his way through dark times is diminished or non-existent. The same is true of memory function. Those tapes that run inside our head—positive thoughts, attitudes, moods and memories, do not function properly. It takes energy to think, to concentrate, and to decide things.

Just like with the automobile, a process exists in the body to re-energize the brain and keep those electrical impulses moving properly and sufficiently along those nerve fibers. That process involves neurotransmitter reuptake.

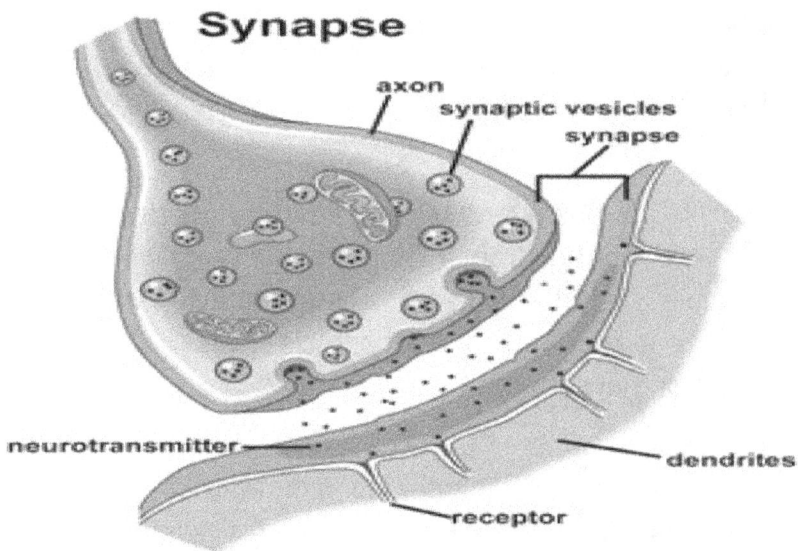

Figure 3: Neurotransmitters and Synapses

Pictured in Figure 3 are two nerve fibers. Nerves are not body length. A nerve for the large toe is not one long nerve fiber. It is a series of cells and fibers extending from the brain to the toe. (Figure 4)

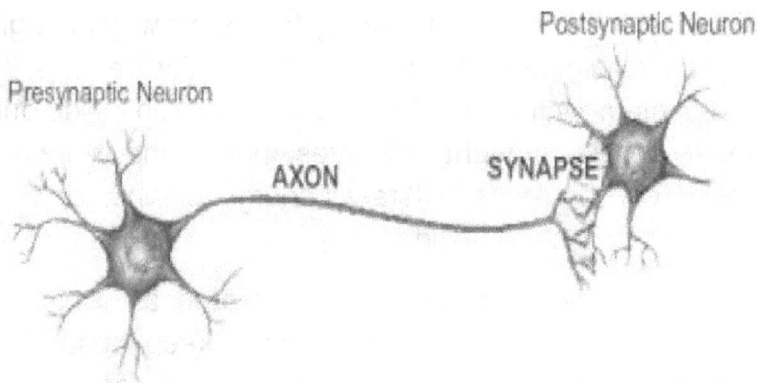

Figure 4: 2 Nerve Cells with Nerve Fibers and Synapse

At one end of a fiber are the neurons that release the hormonal neurotransmitters. At the other end sits the neurotransmitter uptake. Neurotransmitters move between one nerve ending and another. We call this gap between fibers a synapse.

Neurotransmitters pick up energy impulses from one nerve fiber and transmit them to the next one. Eventually, neurotransmitters wear out and depart from the synapse by means of a receptacle. However, with depression new neurotransmitters fail to discharge into the synapse.

The result is that a depletion of neurotransmitters occurs. Insufficient numbers of them are available to pick up the chemical impulses from one nerve fiber and transmit them to the next. Body function is impaired.

Just as the alternator returns energy to the battery, the reuptake of neurotransmitters in the nerve endings recover, restore and redeposit the neurotransmitters into the synapse.

Figure 5 is a substitution of the automotive electrical system by the body's transmission of chemical energy. It shows how the body's electrical impulses work in the body.

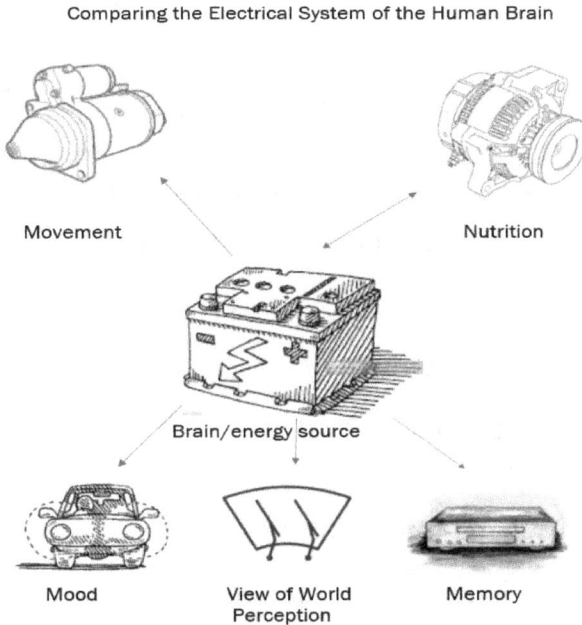

Comparing the Electrical System of the Human Brain

Movement

Nutrition

Brain/energy source

Mood

View of World Perception

Memory

Figure 5: Brain's Electrical System

SUMMARY

When a person has depression, the brain energy level depletes or diminishes. A neurotransmitter is a chemical substance that released at the end of a nerve fiber by the arrival of a nerve impulse and, by diffusing across the synapse or junction, causes the transfer of the impulse to another nerve fiber, a muscle fiber, or some other structure. It transmits signals across a chemical synapse, such as a neuromuscular junction, from one neuron (nerve cell) to another "target" neuron, muscle cell, or gland cell. Nerve fibers release neurotransmitters from synaptic vesicles in synapses into the synaptic cleft and received by receptors on the target cells.

A diagnostic process is necessary to determine exactly what is wrong. Mechanics and clinicians should be wary of a customer or client's word for what is wrong. Such "self-diagnosis" can be misleading and very incorrect. Depleted or inadequate energy impulses, identified as neurotransmitters, affect one's ability to move, think, and see the world in a positive manner.

REVIEW QUESTIONS

(written or discussion)

1. When a person has depression, the brain energy level may be _____.

2. T F A neurotransmitter is a chemical substance.

3. Name 4 types of neurotransmitters.

4. T F Neurotransmitters transfer nerve impulses from one nerve fiber to the next.

5. Neurotransmitters carry impulses from one nerve fiber to another within a gap known as a _____.

6. T F A clinician should take a client's word for what is wrong because the client know what he or she is experiencing.

7. T F A diagnostic process is important in the treatment of depression.

8. One's mood is dependent upon one's chemical energy in the brain.

CLASS DISCUSSION

Why is a good assessment necessary for the diagnosis and treatment of depression? What information should one report in a good assessment? What are warning signal indicates the need for immediate intervention?

Having depression and anxiety at the same time is when you think that your torture will never end and your thoughts about suicide is (sic) unstoppable but you cant kill yourself because you are too scared and afraid as hell and you just hurt yourself, when you wanna (sic) communicate with people but you are so antisocial, when you are dying inside, when you are trying so hard to sleep but end up with crying and over thinking.

-Elizabeth

4

Causes Of Depression

Perplexity abounds regarding the cause or causes of depression. For many observers, depression is not real. These people see others as just "being weak," lazy, or hypochondriac.

For these observers, the seemingly depressed person could and should "just snap out of it." They often think that depressed people are only exaggerating conditions that we all go through from time to time. Depression is merely "manipulation" on the part of the individual.

Sadly, these thoughts and attitudes are incorrect and can be detrimental to the person who is suffering from depression. Depression is real. Depression is painful to the person who experiences it.

CAUSAL FACTORS

So, what causes depression? The answer is neither simple nor is it fully understood. Medical and mental health scientists and practitioners have come far in the understanding of depression and its causes.

Yet we have much remaining to learn. To date, we think there are four known causes of depression. These causes categorize into biological differences, brain chemistry, inherited traits, and life events. To put this in another way, emotional upset, physical trauma, or genetic mutation may cause depression.

Neil Nedley, MD[7], medical director of the Weimar Center of Health and Education, Weimar, California identifies the following causes for depression:

1. Lifestyle – the body needs to be outdoors and to regularly exercise

2. Circadian rhythm – the regulated sleep wake cycle. Early to bed, early to rise seems more than just a saying.

3. Nutrition--Food turns into neurotransmitters

4. Addicting hits including alcoholism, drugs, gambling, and pornography

5. Medical profile including the thyroid

6. Social situations

7. Dr. Nedley strongly advocates for a whole foods, vegetarian diet and sufficient exercise as a major component of treatment. Dr. Nedley also describes certain activities in the frontal lobe of the brain as cause for depression.

8. Frontal lobe causes may include analytical and spiritual processes, circulation, rapid scene activity such as television, the rock music beat, rapid movement as in video games and video music clips

---

7   Nedley, N. (CEO and Medical Director). (2014, May 29). *It Is Written* [Television Broadcast]. Chattanooga. Host: John Bradshaw.

and a lack of Scripture. (Dr. Nedley is a Christian physician.)[8]

According to Dr. Nedley, all these things are bits and pieces related to activity that makes us happy, positive, and hopeful. Others disagree.

Emotional and Lifestyle Causes

Key common emotions may trigger depression. Among them are anger, fear, and guilt. These heavy hitters remain some of the more common emotional causes found in life events.

Anger is a human emotion. Anger occurs when our desires and goals are blocked, when we feel threatened, attacked, frustrated, powerless or embarrassed. Feelings of anger arise due to how one interprets and reacts to certain situations. Everyone has his or her own triggers for what causes anger.

Fear can be deadly. Intense, long occurring and unresolved fear keeps the body in a "fight or flight mode." The body continually prepares to stand up to fearful events or situations or to run from them.

Guilt, more than just a religious construct about sin and redemption, reminds us of past wrongdoing and of unresolved issues. It matters not if reasons actually exist for feelings of guilt. The emotional responses we display because of guilty feelings can cause depression.

In these and other emotions, body changes occur that upset the homeostasis of the body chemistry. With fear, for instance, the body continually produces

---

8   ibid.

adrenalin to provide the necessary energy to fight or to run away. Ongoing fear means ongoing production of excessive adrenalin with which the brain and body must cope.

In this situation, the body attempts to spend off the extra adrenalin by causing body movement. We usually call these "the jitters." The bouncing of the knee while sitting, pacing the floor when nervous or anxious, or even twiddling one's thumbs are ways the body burns off that excess adrenalin.

In much the same way, an angry response requires additional energy. Anger causes the body to react by producing more of the chemical energy to cope with the situation. The greater the anger, the longer the body chemistry is out of balance. When the body chemistry is greatly imbalanced, full-blown rage may occur.

When this energy expends, the body becomes depleted and exhausted. That depletion causes the depressed individual to have insufficient energy for further physical activity or for adequate brain functioning. Hence, the person appears "lazy, indifferent, disinterested, or withdrawn." Severely decreased brain function can look like Alzheimer's disease or other forms of dementia.

Another life-style cause of depression is inadequate nutrition. As we have mentioned, the brain uses chemicals to cause the various body functions. We know that our bodies comprise of a multitude of chemicals, vitamins, hormones, minerals, and water. Our body gets these various nutrients from the foods we eat and the supplements we take.

Proper nutrition, adequate digestion, and physical exercise are important for a fully functional body. Lifestyle changes may be necessary in nutrition and physical activity in order for the body to function at its peak. For this reason, nutritional and physical activity assessments become useful tools in determining the presence of depression.

Biological Causes and Hormones

What are hormones? Hormones are chemical substances produced in an organism and transported in tissue fluids such as blood or sap to stimulate and regulate substance specific cells or tissues into action. A hormone may be a synthetic substance with an effect similar to that of an animal or plant hormone. Both cortical and sex hormones exist. Researchers think that a person's sex hormones influence behavior or mood.

Peptide hormones are water-soluble hormones comprised of a few amino acids that introduce multiple series of chemical reactions to change a cell's metabolism. Examples include hormones of the pituitary gland and the parathyroid glands. Small peptide hormones include thyrotropin-releasing hormone (TRH) and vasopressin.

Unlike steroid hormones, which can cross through a cell's membrane and enter the cell, peptide hormones cannot pass through the membrane. Instead, peptide hormones bind to receptors on the outside of cells, which triggers a response inside the cell.

We refer to Peptides, composed of scores or hundreds of amino acids, as proteins. Examples of protein hormones include insulin and growth hormone. More complex protein hormones bear carbohydrate side-chains called glycoprotein hormones.

Protein hormones are similar to peptide hormones. They have longer amino acid chain lengths than the peptides. These hormones have an effect on the endocrine system of animals, including humans.

Protein hormones are a type of chemical compound in the body that regulates metabolism and cell function. They are derived from amino acids (the building blocks of proteins) and facilitate signaling between cells of the endocrine system and various other cells of the body.

A steroid hormone is a steroid that acts as a hormone. Steroid hormones group into two classes: corticosteroids (typically made in the adrenal cortex, hence cortico-) and sex steroids (typically made in the gonads or placenta). They have some of the characteristics of true steroids as receptor ligands.

Most lipid hormones derive from cholesterol, so they are structurally similar to it. Examples of steroid hormones include estradiol, which is an estrogen, or female sex hormone, and testosterone, which is an androgen, or male sex hormone. The above provides only an overview of hormones, not considered extensive or complete.

Brain Chemistry

As we have noted, the chemical make up of the brain has significant impact on the body. The brain converts various chemicals into energy impulses that transmit throughout the body. The brain depends on glands in the body to produce the chemicals required. A delicate balance exists in the body chemistry of the brain.

Read more about brain chemistry and hormones in Chapter 9.

Physical Causes: Stress and Trauma

Hormone changes may occur for a variety of reasons. Physical stress and trauma are two of those reasons. Here is an example related to physical trauma.

The author recounts this example of a physical trauma, which caused depression in a teenager, the cause misdiagnosed by a highly competent inpatient clinical staff of nurses, psychological examiner, and social worker trained in emotional and psychological aspects of the disorder.

Mason was a 17-year-old high school senior. He owned a new truck, which he was driving with his best friend Scott in the passenger seat. At the time, seatbelts requirements did not include trucks. As Mason drove through an intersection, having the right of way, another vehicle struck his truck on the passenger side door. The impact threw Scott into the windshield with such force that Scott's neck was immediately broken.

Mason also bounced against the frame of the truck's cab, fracturing four ribs and breaking his right leg just above the ankle. The police found that Mason was in no way at fault, having the right of way, driving within the speed limit, and obeying all the applicable driving laws.

Within a week, Mason became lethargic, moody, intermittently angry and tearful, and restless. Soon he lost interest in his favorite activities and withdrew from his friends.

When Mason quit eating, his parents decided something needed to happen. His family physician determined that Mason was depressed and referred him to a psychiatrist. The psychiatrist was sufficiently concerned that he hospitalized Mason in a very prominent local hospital that had a 28-bed inpatient acute care psychiatric unit.

Staff completed a nursing assessment, a battery of psychological diagnostic tests, activity therapy assessment, nutritional assessment, and a full social history. The hospital staff determined that Mason would benefit from a regimen of therapeutic medications, participation in daily classes to help Mason understand himself and his depression, and daily psychological counseling. He would also benefit from structured crafts and physical activities that accommodated his broken ribs and ankle.

The staff met with the psychiatrist and proposed a treatment plan based on the various assessments. The doctor rejected the plan of care and said Mason did not need all those interventions, although he did agree with the dietary plan recommended by the nutritionist.

When the author came to the hospital as the new director of the inpatient unit, he encountered complete controversial concerns by the hospital staff about the treatment plan ordered by the psychiatrist.

One by one the Charge Nurse, the Psychological Examiner, the Clinical Social Worker, and the Activities Therapist raised their concerns and objections. The author listened patiently and with some empathy to the presentations of the staff. The author, as both the director of the unit and the clinical chief, decided to interview Mason. The staff attended the interview with the condition they neither comment nor question Mason during that time.

"Tell me what's going on with you and your depression," the author said. Mason looked up from the floor, making the first significant eye contact with any staff member since his admission. "I know I am depressed. I know things are not right. But, I don't think it as bad as it seems."

"What do you mean by that? Tell me more," the author calmly said. "Everyone seems to think that I am depressed because I killed my best friend. That's just not true. I know Scott was killed in the accident. I know the accident was not my fault. I really don't feel guilty about being responsible for his death. I feel sad. I wish it hadn't happened. But I didn't do anything wrong and I could not have prevented the accident. But everyone thinks I feel guilty. They want me to talk about my guilt feelings. They try to occupy my mind with crafts. And I have to sit in these classes about how to deal with my stress, anger and guilt. That's not me."

After a few more minutes, the interview concluded, staff assisted Mason back to his room. The staff seemed puzzled and in disbelief. However, none admitted to having talked to Mason about how he was thinking about his life at that moment. They only focused on his "guilt."

The Director concurred with the psychiatrist and kept Mason from participating in the proposed treatment plan. He consulted with the psychiatrist and it was determined the staff, a very competent one with lots of experience and skill, needed some in-service education on the topic.

At the next treatment planning staff meeting, the psychiatrist taught the staff about how physical trauma might cause depression—a new concept for the staff. Because of the trauma, Mason's body chemistry had significantly altered in order to adapt to the physical condition. This had caused his depression.

Physical trauma has a great impact on one's emotional state. Here is another example.

Myrtle took pride and consolation in her ability to live independently in her home of 57 years. Although her husband had been deceased for 15 years, Myrtle had a happy and active life with friends, the Women's Club, her church, and family. Myrtle also enjoyed good health for her age—80 years.

One afternoon, Myrtle fell and experienced intense pain in her left hip. Using her medical alert system, she was able to call for assistance. The paramedics transported her to a local emergency room.

Upon examination and x-rays, Myrtle was told that she had a broken hip. As she lived alone, the emergency room physician determined that Myrtle needed to stay in a nursing facility for recovery and physical therapy. Although not happy with this option, Myrtle accepted the decision.

Soon, Myrtle was showing signs of mild depression. Her friends began to whisper, "She fell and broke her hip. She thinks she will be unable to live independently after this. I don't blame her for getting depressed, Nursing homes are no fun. People die in nursing homes."

The facts, however, disputed what her friends were saying. First, Myrtle did not fall and break her leg. As in most cases with the elderly, the hip broke and caused Myrtle to fall. Her weakened and somewhat brittle bones could not bear up any longer.

Furthermore, Myrtle had no thoughts or fears of losing her independence. She was still hopeful for her future life. However, the trauma and shock of the broken bone and the body's natural response to it caused that critical shift in Myrtle's hormonal balance.

Genetics and Inherited Traits

One of the most exciting areas in our consideration of the causes of depression is the area of genetics and inherited traits. Scientific breakthroughs in the study of genetics have revealed some interesting possibilities for further consideration. Yet this controversial research needs more study, testing, and examination.

Some scientists point to a specific gene, identified as C4, as a cause of depression, bi-polar disorder, and schizophrenia. The gene appears to have a molecular discrepancy or modification. Other scientists are skeptical that C4 is a sole cause of these disorders.

In disorders such as depression, diabetes, and high blood pressure, a combination of genetic changes seem to predispose some people to become ill. Especially in Major Depressive Disorder, more than one genetic factor may be responsible for the predisposition of certain individuals for the condition. Today, it is very doubtful that any one gene causes depression in any large number of people

We think that depression has an inherited aspect and that it runs in families. If someone has a parent or sibling with major depression, that person probably has a two or three times greater risk of developing depression compared with the average person. Clearly, significant additional research is required to clarify our current understanding of genetics and heredity as causes of depression.

SUMMARY

Causes of depression categorize as biological differences, brain chemistry, emotional upset, physical trauma, and genetic mutation, inherited traits, and life events. Any or a combination of these factors may cause depression. Three key common emotions – anger, fear, and guilt, may trigger depression.

Hormones are chemical substances produced in an organism and transported in tissue fluids such as blood or sap to stimulate and regulate substance specific cells or tissues into action. Glands in the body produce the chemicals required by the brain to create energy impulses. Proper nutrition provides the essential elements of chemistry for creation of the chemistry needed for the brain.

In disorders such as depression, diabetes, and high blood pressure, a combination of genetic changes seem to predispose some people to become ill. Especially in Major Depressive Disorder, more than one genetic factor may be responsible for the predisposition of certain individuals for the condition. Today, it is very doubtful that any one gene causes depression in any large number of people.

REVIEW QUESTIONS
(written or discussion)

1. Name the four known categories of causes of depression.

2. T F Depression may be caused by emotional upset, physical trauma, and genetic mutation.

3. 3 common emotional causes of depression are _____, _____, and _____.

4. How do hormones function in the body?

5. What produces the chemicals used by the brain to create energy impulses?

6. What is the effect of nutrition on whether one develops depression?

7. Is it possible for a broken bone to cause depression?
    Yes No

8. T F Scientists can point to one specific gene that
    determines one's predisposition toward depression.

CLASS DISCUSSION

How might the various potential causes of
depression interact to create the potential for depression
in an individual? To what extent does hormonal change
and brain chemistry affect the symptoms of depression?

5

Persistent Depressive Episode

Depression is a word frequently used by people to describe a condition that few of us truly understand. Depression is not a day or two of sadness, tearfulness, or feeling down. As my friend Jim Gilbertson of Chattanooga, Tennessee says, "We all have days like that."

This is a truthful comment about human emotions and the condition of humankind. Three things you should know about depression:

1. Depression may be more than just an emotional or attitudinal problem

2. Most people don't understand what depression is or how it affects a person

3. Depression may occur more commonly than people think.

Two diagnostic types of depression—Persistent Depressive Disorder and Major Depressive Disorder or clinical depression, exist, although they appear in multiple and varying ways. We will look at an overview of conventional depressive episodes and the forms they take. This overview is a generic one and not considered as an extensive presentation.

NATURE OF PERSISTENT DEPRESSIVE DISORDER

The most commonly known form of depression, also known as Persistent Depressive Disorder—once known as dysthymia or just depression, has a less severe manifestation and more easily responds to treatment. People with this form of depression respond well to medications or to counseling and behavioral changes. This form of treatment commonly has a physical, environmental or emotional cause.

The person with true clinical depression, a psychiatric medical condition, has a condition with multiple symptoms that last for weeks, months, years, or even a lifetime. Depression is a common but serious mood and thought disorder. Depression may cause severe symptoms that affect how you feel, think, and handle daily activities, such as sleeping, eating, or working. For a diagnosis of depression, the symptoms must be present for at least two weeks.

The individual with Persistent Depressive Disorder may find it hard to be upbeat even on happy occasions — he or she may be described as having a gloomy personality, constantly complaining or incapable of having fun. Though Persistent Depressive Disorder is not as severe as major depression, a currently depressed mood may be mild to severe.

Because of the chronic nature of persistent depressive disorder, coping with depression's symptoms can be challenging. A combination of talk therapy and medication can be effective in treating this condition. In many instances a course of behavioral modification may also be beneficial.

Persistent depressive disorder may come and go over a period of years, and its intensity may change over time. Typically, the symptoms of Persistent Depressive Disorder do not disappear for more than two months at a time. In addition, major depression episodes may occur before or during Persistent Depressive Disorder sometimes called double depression.

The *exact* cause of Persistent Depressive Disorder remains not known. In fact, more than one causal factor may be involved. These factors include biological differences, brain chemistry, inherited traits, and life events discussed in Chapter 4.

Persistent Depressive Disorder is more prevalent in women than in men. Estimates indicate that as much as 4% of the population has Persistent Depressive Disorder. It can begin in childhood or in adulthood. It can be difficult to detect.

Persistent Depressive Disorder may be characterized by dysphoria--a state of unease or generalized dissatisfaction with life. It may also be characterized by its persistence—persisting for at least two years or more. Sadly, studies suggest a substantial proportion of sufferers do not experience a sustained recovery.

Persistent depressive disorder presents as characterized by an insidious onset, waxing and waning symptoms of at least two years duration, and possibly brief periods of normal mood. In contrast, major depression characterizes by a fairly well defined onset, sustained symptoms, and discrete episodes. Most primary care clinicians are fairly well-trained in the detection and diagnosis of major depression. This is likely because the symptoms of major depression are more dramatic and oftentimes anchored around identifiable alterations in functions in daily living. Therefore, when patients broach the subject of "depression," many clinicians promptly cue to their mental templates for major depression, unintentionally overlooking the diagnosis of dysthymic disorder. This phenomenon may also occur in mental health settings.

Health care professionals would do well to probe into the individual who experiences mood, attitudinal, cognitive, and physical symptoms. Take care to listen attentively to every expression of dissatisfaction or dysfunction more clearly to understand the symptoms and conditions experienced by the individual. A comprehensive social history is mandatory.

Family members frequently go into a clinician's office reporting that the concerned individual is depressed, or losing his mind, or some other form of "diagnosis," which is merely an expression of an opinion. Family should refrain from these suggestions, even if well intended to give the clinician some clue about the individual's condition. Such a process may set the process of diagnosis off the track.

Several instances of Major Depressive Disorder have occurred and determined to be Alzheimer's disease because a clear explanation of what was occurring in the individual's live was not forthcoming. The best course of action by family members is simply to describe the individual's behavior and physical appearance.

"He just seemed to stop caring for his personal hygiene." "He stopped shaving." "She has quit eating." "He loves to fish but doesn't go out with his fishing buddies any longer." "He seems not to concentrate on things like he once did." "She doesn't seem to remember things like she should." "He soils himself all the time."

These types of statements help the clinician assess what might be going on with the individual. Too often, a family member notices the individual having problems with memory or concentration, or decision-making. An immediate assumption is the person developed Alzheimer's.

It may be just a case of severe depression. Clear descriptions of behavior, troublesome conversations, and physical appearance make for a better assessment. The clinician needs and seeks that information.

One thing more. If the individual experiences difficulty in answering the clinician's questions or gives a wrong answer, family members should not prompt the individual, correct her, or answer for him. The clinician is not "testing" the individual. The clinician is not looking for a correct answer. Rather the clinician is looking at cognitive functioning to determine the severity of the dysfunction.

DIAGNOSTIC CRITERIA FOR PERSISTENT DEPRESSIVE DISORDER DSM-5th Edition

1. Depressed mood for most of the day, for more days than not, as indicated by either subjective account or observation by others, for at least 2 years. Note: In children and adolescents, mood

can be irritable and duration must be at least 1
year.

2. Presence, while depressed, of two (or more) of the
    following:

    a. Poor appetite or overeating.

    b. Insomnia or hypersomnia.

    c. Low energy or fatigue.

    d. Low self-esteem.

    e. Poor concentration or difficulty making
        decisions.

    f. Feelings of hopelessness.

3. During the 2-year period (1 year for children or
    adolescents) of the disturbance, the individual has
    never been without the symptoms in Criteria A and
    B for more than 2 months at a time.

4. Criteria for a major depressive disorder may be
    continuously present for 2 years.

5. There has never been a manic episode or a
    hypomanic episode, and criteria have never been
    met for cyclothymic disorder.

6. The disturbance is not better explained by a
    persistent schizoaffective disorder, schizophrenia,
    delusional disorder, or other specified or
    unspecified schizophrenia spectrum and other
    psychotic disorder.

7. The symptoms are not attributable to the
    physiological effects of a substance (e.g., a drug of

abuse, a medication) or another medical condition (e.g., hypothyroidism).

8. The symptoms cause clinically significant distress or impairment in social, occupational, or other important areas of functioning.

9. **Note:** Because the criteria for a major depressive episode include four symptoms that are absent from the symptom list for persistent depressive disorder (dysthymia), a very limited number of individuals will have depressive symptoms that have persisted longer than 2 years but will not meet criteria for persistent depressive disorder. If full criteria for a major depressive episode have been met at some point during the current episode of illness, they should be given a diagnosis of major depressive disorder. Otherwise, a diagnosis of other specified depressive disorder or unspecified depressive disorder is warranted.

SUMMARY

Depression may be more than just an emotional or attitudinal problem. Two diagnostic types of depression— persistent depressive disorder and Major Depressive Disorder or clinical depression, exist, although they appear in multiple and varying ways.

The exact cause of Persistent Depressive Disorder is not known. In fact, more than one causal factor may be involved. These factors include biological differences, brain chemistry, inherited traits, and life events. It occurs more frequently in women than in men and may affect a person of any age, from childhood to old age.

Depression may go undiagnosed or misdiagnosed due to lack of clear and sufficient information about a patient's behavior. A comprehensive social history or clinical assessment assists the physician in making an accurate differential diagnosis of the patient's condition.

REVIEW QUESTIONS

(written or discussion)

1. T F Persistent depressive disorder is merely an attitudinal or emotional condition.
2. Name two diagnostic types of depression.
3. Name the less severe form of depression.
4. T F Behavioral change (behavior modification) may be an effective way of treating Persistent depressive disorder.
5. What are four causal factors for depression?
6. What is double depression?
7. T F Women experience Persistent Depressive Disorder more often than do men.
8. T F As much as 4% of the population has a dysthymic disorder.
9. Define dysphoria.
10. T. F Persistent Depressive Disorder may be overlooked or misdiagnosed.

CLASS DISCUSSION

How does a Persistent Depressive Disorder affect an individual? What domains of function does it affect? What causes depression?

6

Major Depressive Disorder

CLINICAL DEPRESSION

Depression does not go away for everyone. For many people, depression is temporary and passes without intervention or once the person has expressed the feelings and resolved the thoughts causing the depression. However, a small percentage of people remain who can talk about their issues, express their feelings, take very good care of themselves emotionally, even take medication and have a great life, and still be depressed throughout their lives.

These individuals may have periods of feeling good, periods of feeling less bad, and periods of feeling horrible—for these people, their depression never goes away permanently. To people around them, these individuals seem healthy and alive. Deep inside, however, the struggle to survive cognitively and emotionally is intense.

DEPRESSION VERSUS MAJOR DEPRESSION

Depression and major depression, also known as clinical depression, are actually different things, and they produce different symptoms. With major depression, it can be difficult to work, study, sleep, eat and enjoy activities with friends and family. Clinical depression can affect people only once in their life, and it can affect others several times in a lifetime.

Major depression can occur from one generation to the next in different families, but it can also affect people with no family history of the illness. It is common for people to feel sad at some point in their lives. However, if symptoms persist every day for at least two weeks, it can be a sign of clinical depression.

Major depressive disorder is the medical term for repeated episodes of a very intense, deep depression that is disabling and enormously painful. People commonly known as bipolar may experience similar disabling depression during their depressive phases. Often between episodes, people return to a functional, happy state. Sometimes people can also have a milder depression, even between episodes of major depression.

Some people experience "atypical" depression. They can be in a deep depressive episode and yet appear to come out of it long enough to laugh or enjoy something briefly before sinking back in, or can act normal for short periods of time or during certain activities. This can be confusing for both the depressed individual and to others around them.

This condition is not an indication that the person is any less depressed or any less in danger than someone found in a major depressive episode that does not have those brief breaks. It is just depression in a different form. Atypical depression characterizes by feeling emotionally paralyzed, physically leaden— barely able to move or engage in any activity, and often overeating, oversleeping, or experiencing some sensitivity to rejection.

NATURE OF MAJOR DEPRESSIVE DISORDER

Most people find difficulty in under-standing deeper forms of depression. Looking at people with illnesses or injuries usually means individuals see runny noses, blood, high temperatures, or fractures. What one sees in a person with depression are lethargy, crying and sadness, irritability, and hostility. They see an individual expressing helplessness and hopelessness. They just need to "buck up."

We associate these behaviors with personality and moral character. We think people choose to be the way they are. We seldom see these as symptoms of an illness that has taken over the person's personality.

Most of us wonder why the continually depressed person does not just get over it and may even wonder whether it is a manipulation. We think the person is just lazy, weak, or giving in to something, which he or she could fight. Yet the person who experiences this depression can find it difficult to explain because it is extremely painful in ways for which words fail; and it generalizes throughout the body rather than identified in a specific part of the body such as would be the case with a cut arm, for instance.

People with chronic, severe depression are not gratifying or indulging themselves. They are not lazy, manipulating, or exaggerating their pain and dysfunction. They are not giving in to a condition that they should be able to resist.

Although this kind of depression – clinically described as an illness, in comparison to other debilitating, painful, potentially fatal illnesses or injuries, severe depression is unique in how it affects one's mind, behavior, personality, and thought processes. Because the mind is part of the illness, people usually do not see the dynamics of this debilitating and paralyzing condition. Exasperation, resentment or animosity can override any notions of patience and empathy.

Successive major depressive episodes make it more certain that additional episodes will occur. Statistically, we know that each episode increases the probability other episodes are likely and with increased frequency. It is also likely that during hormonal situations such as menstruation, pregnancy, childbirth, perimeno-pause, and menopause, woman with major depression likely will be at greater risk of having still another episode.

OTHER FORMS OF DEPRESSION

Some forms of depression appear as slightly different, or they may develop under unique circumstances, such as:

Perinatal depression is much more serious than the "baby blues," those relatively mild depressive and anxiety symptoms that typically clear within two weeks after delivery that many women experience after giving birth. Women with perinatal depression experience full-blown major depression during pregnancy or after delivery (postpartum depression). The feelings of extreme sadness, anxiety, and exhaustion that accompany perinatal depression may make it difficult for these new mothers to complete daily care activities for themselves and/or for their babies. These depressions may be largely because of hormonal shifts in the body chemistry of these women.

Psychotic depression occurs when a person has severe depression plus some form of psychosis, such as having disturbing false fixed beliefs (delusions) or hearing or seeing upsetting things that others cannot hear or see (hallucinations). The psychotic symptoms typically have a depressive "theme," such as delusions of guilt, poverty, or illness. Sadly, we many times overlook the depressive features of these psychoses and they go untreated. The treating physician requires full information to treat adequately the condition.

Seasonal Affective Disorder occurs as the onset of depression during the winter months, when there is less natural sunlight. This depression generally lifts during spring and summer. Winter depression, accompanied typically by social withdrawal, increased sleep, and weight gain, predictably returns every year in seasonal affective disorder.

Cyclothymic Disorder (once known as Manic Depression and later as Bi-Polar Disorder) is different from depression, but it is included in this list because someone with Cyclothymic Disorder experiences episodes of extremely low moods that meet the criteria for major depression (called "bipolar depression"). Nevertheless, a person with Cyclothymic Disorder may also experiences extreme high – euphoric or irritable, moods called "mania" or a less severe form called "hypomania."

According to the National Institute of Mental Health (NIMH), examples of other types of depressive disorders newly added to the diagnostic classification of DSM-5 include disruptive mood dysregulation disorder (diagnosed in children and adolescents) and premenstrual dysphoric disorder (PMDD).

DIAGNOSTIC CRITERIA FOR MAJOR DEPRESSIVE DISORDER DSM-5th Edition

A. Five (or more) of the following symptoms have been present during the same 2-week period and represent a change from previous functioning; at least one of the symptoms is either (1) depressed mood or (2) loss of interest or pleasure.

Note: Do not include symptoms that are clearly attributable to another medical condition.

1. Depressed mood most of the day, nearly every day, as indicated by either subjective report (e.g., feels sad, empty, hopeless) or observation made by others (e.g., appears tearful). Note: In children and adolescents, can be irritable mood.

2. Markedly diminished interest or pleasure in all, or almost all, activities most of the day, nearly every day (as indicated by either subjective account or observation)

3. Significant weight loss when not dieting or weight gain (e.g., a change of more than 5% of body weight in a month), or decrease or increase in appetite nearly every day. Note:

In children, consider failure to make expected weight gain.

4. Insomnia or hypersomnia nearly every day

5. Psychomotor agitation or retardation nearly every day (observable by others, not merely subjective feelings of restlessness or of being slowed down)

6. Fatigue or loss of energy nearly every day

7. Feelings of worthlessness or excessive or inappropriate guilt (which may be delusional) nearly every day (not merely self-reproach or guilt about being sick)

8. Diminished ability to think or concentrate, or indecisiveness, nearly every day (either by subjective account or as observed by others)

9. Recurrent thoughts of death (not just fear of dying), recurrent suicidal ideation without a specific plan, or a suicide attempt or a specific plan for committing suicide

B. The symptoms cause clinically significant distress or impairment in social, occupational, or other important areas of functioning.

C. The episode is not attributable to the physiological effects of a substance or to another medical condition.

Note: Criteria A-C represent a major depressive episode

Note: Responses to a significant loss (e.g., bereavement, financial ruin, losses from a natural disaster, a serious medical illness or disability) may include the feelings of intense sadness, rumination about the loss, insomnia, poor appetite, and weight loss noted in Criterion A, which may resemble a depressive episode. Although such symptoms may be understandable or considered appropriate to the loss, the presence of a major depressive episode in addition to the normal response to a significant loss should also be carefully considered. This decision inevitably requires the exercise of clinical judgment based on the individual's history and the cultural norms for the expression of distress in the contest of loss.

The occurrence of the major depressive episode is not better explained by schizoaffective disorder, schizophrenia, schizophreniform disorder, delusional disorder, or other specified and unspecified schizophrenia spectrum and other psychotic disorders.

SUMMARY

Depression does not go away for everyone. A small percentage of people remain who can talk about their issues, express their feelings, take very good care of themselves emotionally, even take medication and have a great life, and still be depressed throughout their lives. To people around them, these individuals seem healthy and alive even while struggling deep inside. The hope remains that even this type of depression remains treatable. A meaningful life may occur.

Because the mind is part of the illness, people usually do not see the dynamics of this debilitating and paralyzing condition. Exasperation, resentment or animosity can override any notions of patience and empathy. Successive major depressive episodes make it more certain that additional episodes will occur.

In comparison to other debilitating, painful, potentially fatal illnesses or injuries, severe depression is unique in how it affects one's mind, behavior, personality, and thought processes. Some other forms of depression include perinatal depression, seasonal affective disorder, psychotic depression, and cyclothymic disorder. Examples of other types of depressive disorders newly added to the diagnostic classification of DSM-5 include disruptive mood dysregulation disorder (diagnosed in children and adolescents) and premenstrual dysphoric disorder (PMDD).

REVIEW QUESTIONS

(written or discussion)

1. What is a major depressive disorder?

2. How does a Major Depressive Disorder differ from a persistent depressive disorder?

3. How are Persistent Depressive Disorder and Major Depressive Disorder alike?

4. T F   Major Depression can be a debilitating and paralyzing condition.

CLASS DISCUSSION

How does a person live with a chronic disability that cannot be effectively described to those around them? How do people function? How do loved ones take care of them long-term? How do relationships survive?

7

The Face Of Depression

THE REAL STUFF

Now our study comes to the transition from the academic to the experiential. In this chapter, comments from individuals on social media present an actual view of how depressed individuals think and how they feel. This is "the real stuff," from people actually in the throes of depressive episodes.

The format of this presentation on depression shifts in this chapter. Rather than having topics for class discussion at the end of the chapter, discussion will occur throughout the chapter regarding the material presented. The learner can consider this a case study of a type.

These case study examples are actual comments by real patients. Some of the posts are from social media postings. We identify the depressed person as James. However, the examples are from several individual clients.

These case examples will cover topical areas such as anger, motivation, decision-making, energy, stress, negativity, emotional, initiative, whining, a cry for help, cognition, and discouragement—all of which relate to depression. In class discussion, identify those areas, traits, and symptoms that seem associated with the case examples. What is James actually saying or asking? Discuss what interventions might work. Are the examples ones that everyone experiences? How might they be different from what people without depression experience?

1. Growing up, I was never allowed to express that I was angry. I was not allowed to discuss my anger. I was not allowed to show anger toward my parents. Authority was authority. To do so was to exacerbate the situation. To express anger or an opinion of my own created more anger and repercussions toward me. Feelings could be hurt if I didn't agree with the company line. So I internalized all that anger. By age 14 all that rage created a life long major depression. Coming to terms with it has been a struggle. Now, I find myself in a similar circumstance. More than frustrated, more than upset, I am angry and I am not able to express it without causing return anger and hurt feelings. And that makes me angry. I'm stuck in something I don't yet know how to resolve. I'm trying to sin not in my anger and not going to bed angry. So far I have not sinned--that I know of, but I have had about 2 weeks of sleepless nights, stressed out body systems, and cognitive paralysis that has blocked completion of a project. A lot is going on.

2. I am out of two medications--one for diabetes and one for sleep apnea/depression. Refills are ready. Pharmacy is 8 minutes away. It's a beautiful sunny day, warm and pleasant. All I need to do is get in the car and go get it. And I am struggling with that chore--yes, I said chore. For you it is a simple thing. For me it is a major event. Don't give me all you sage advice and motivational statements. I already know all that.

It isn't easy for depressives, despite what you think. Your world is not colored the same way as mine, and neither of us can change that.

3. I'm sitting in a chair in the living room, in front of the TV. I have my cell phone in one hand and my dinner plate in the other. I want to put the plate on the ottoman in front of the chair, but it has a lot of clutter on it. I have spent 5 minutes trying to figure out where to put the cell phone in order to free up one hand to clear away the clutter on the ottoman. I really don't know what to do. OK. I figured out where to put the phone so I could place the tray on the ottoman. I ate my dinner and now I'm up, brushing my teeth and taking bedtime medications. I know many if you think I was silly in not knowing where to put the phone. But see, that's a reflection of impaired decision making. Simple things become difficult.

4. (This is a different case from #3 just above.) Finished dinner. Sitting in a chair in the living room. Need to get up. Telling my brain that I need to get up. The energy is not flowing. Need to put the tray on the foot stool so I can stand. Just can't decide to do it. I'm really conflicted. Just stand up, James. This is another face of depression.

5. March: 12 continuous days of diarrhea, flat tire, increasing periodic depression, four days of muscle pain, broken car seat--story of my life. Most likely. Weakened but not defeated. That's why it is important to have Christian friends joining in the battle. Thank you Christian friends. Your prayers and comments of a Spiritual nature, rather than those of the secular

"human nature," help win the battle with your encouragement and not criticism. You are the Spirit's vessel in this warfare. I love you all. The victory is The Lord's and you are His hands, feet, mouth, and fingers. This is how the body of Christ functions.

6. People like to play word games. This makes me both sad and angry. Their attempts at profundity sicken me. It's just a smokescreen to, as you say, pretend to care but don't. You are spot on, Bobby. Don't let them distract or divert the dialog.

7. To those of you reaching out in support know that those of us in depression are dominated usually by emotional stuff, and all the cognitive and logic just pass us by. Take action. Go there, not ask us to come where you are.

8. I had a graduate professor of whom it was said he could step over dozens of starving children to fight the causes of hunger. So while it is important to educate "them," someone needs to be actively intervening with "us." Your words to "assure us" don't. Come over and pick me up and take me where you want me to go. If you are waiting for me to get out of the residence and meet you somewhere by my own initiative, it will most probably never happen. You don't understand this? You probably don't understand depression as well as you think you do.

9. Depression. Yeah, I know. You've heard it all before. But I want to say that you told me more than once to stop whining. I wasn't ventilating per se, although there was a lot of that. You said you also had been depressed but got over it. That wasn't helpful in the

least. I wasn't explaining and educating, although there was an element of that. So, why then did I expose my soul to you on Facebook©? Here is the hard part, and I apologize in advance if anyone is offended. I was talking mostly to what little family I have left and some church friends. I was crying out for help. I was seeking someone to intervene in my deepest gloom and fear as I tumbled deeper toward suicide. It took everything in me, and my trust in God, to stay alive. No one took the time, effort, or energy to get involved. No one came to check on me. What I got was lectures, platitudes, some expressions of sympathy, shared experiences, and criticism. Some words of support. But no intervention. Where was my family? Where was the church? Who in the Body came to spend some time? No one. Absolutely no one. "Well, you know I this or that," or "I would have but..." several possible scenarios in March. First of all, I did warn of it's coming back in February. Now my postings in March were actually not whining, although I was told so by more than one person.

10. I was seen for depression first time in 1958. My first meds for depression were in 1977. I was diagnosed with major depression in 1990s. Had an industrial accident in 1999 and diagnosed with PTSD. Shabbily treated by workers compensation, I have not been fully paid or reimbursed for out of pocket expenses. The case is still in litigation and I can't get my paperwork done. That task is overwhelming me. I can't organize the material. I can't focus. I get bored and distracted trying to complete the paperwork. I

can't decide where to start or how to break through the impasse.

11. I get so discouraged. I am not suicidal but I do think about it. I'm just afraid to try it. And who would take care of my wonderful dog that I promised to care for. I am religious but have little trust in the Christian community. Most everyone fails to understand my depression and PTSD and just give me the usual "get over it" platitudes. I have been in most of the mental health facilities in my community and don't really feel comfortable returning there for help, mostly because I never got better. I just received their "treatment program" that was "tailored to my depression" but not for major depression with physical medical issues. No clinical person I have ever dealt with seems to grasp the difference in treatment for depression and major depression. And there were no practical daily living interventions to ease the burdens.

12. When I have sought help or some kind of encouragement from my friends (my family don't really seem to care), I know they mean well with their "advice." They tell me to stay hydrated, to drink lots of water. They say I need to make myself exercise more. I am reminded that "we all go through these problems." I'm told I just need to make myself. I should reach out. I should get involved helping someone less fortunate and see how good I have it. I should eat better meals and cut out on the potatoes, pastas, breads, sweets, and rice. But that's the bulk of what I receive each month from the community food pantry. Anyway, I get angry because I already know all that. It's like these people think I am ignorant and they

need to inform me of a better way. I don't need that kind of help. I need physical contact with a human being. I sit at home for days on end, never receiving a telephone call or a personal text. If someone were to actually come over and take me out to eat or to see a movie or go shopping for groceries, I would pass out from the shock.

How did your discussion go? What have you learned about depression? How has your thinking changed?

SUMMARY

Twelve actual case situations demonstrate the real stuff, the actual description of depressive disorder from the perspective of the one who is depressed. These case studies reflect internalized anger, fear, and guilt—not always obviously displayed. The studies show the hopelessness, the isolation, and the despair of individuals who suffer from a depressive disorder.

The studies provide a critical view of how depression distorts or confuses cognitive processes. A majority of those interacting with a depressed person cannot understand such cognition difficulties. The cry for help often goes unanswered.

T. S. Eliot wrote in 1922 "*The Wasteland*,"

APRIL is the cruelest month, breeding
Lilacs out of the dead land, mixing
Memory and desire, stirring
Dull roots with spring rain.
Winter kept us warm, covering
Earth in forgetful snow, feeding
A little life with dried tubers.

"*Breeding/Lilacs out of the dead land*" is a very heavy, depressed way to describe the blooming of flowers. ... In summary; April is the cruelest month because the life and color of spring throws one's depression into stark relief and forces painful memories to surface.

He sees the same things as everyone else, but there is no joy there. "*Mixing/Memory and desire, stirring/Dull roots with spring rain*"; a sense of loss and longing, of being rooted in the past, and spring re-awakening memories of things that have passed. By comparison; "*Winter kept us warm*" "*forgetful snow*"; these things suggest a state of comfortable emotional hibernation.

A wise literature teacher once put it in this way; when your arm is numb, you don't feel it. But when the blood flows again, with all those the pins and needles, suddenly you know about it. It's not (emotional or depressive) numbness that hurts; it's the return of feeling.

Anyone who has dealt with long-term depression can probably feel the connection to what Eliot is describing here, and it does a fantastic job of leading in to the rest of the poem, which deals excruciatingly with depression and memory.

8

Interview With "James"

Following is an actual interview of "James." Consider what he is telling us in his responses. Then answer the review questions at the end of the chapter.

What was your first sign that something was wrong? What symptoms did you experience?

Sadness. Loneliness, even when I was around friends. I remember it was the year the Platters came out with the song "The Great Pretender." I felt it was really describing me—without the girlfriend love interest. "Yes, I'm the great pretender, pretending that I'm doing well. My need is such I pretend too much. I'm lonely but no one can tell." I didn't feel close to my parents or my siblings. Family relationships were such a struggle. There was a lot of violence in the home.

What was the diagnosis experience like?

Well, that's an interesting question. My diagnostic experience was two-phased. When I first told my mother that I thought I needed to see a psychiatrist, she really got upset and tore into me. My dad was somewhat of a hypochondriac and had a set of medical books that were forbidden for me to read. Dad went through those books, and it seemed like he caught every disease and illness in them, from A to Z in order.

So I remember riding in the car and having my mother telling me "One thing I just can't stand is someone thinking he's sick when he's not." My dad's hypochondria really worked on her a lot. However, she did arrange for me to see a psychiatrist. It was not a good experience for me. I felt very uncomfortable with him.

We talked about depression and some other things, but when I got home, I told my mother that he said there was nothing wrong with me. I just didn't want to go back to him. And I thought the family was having financial trouble and I didn't want to be a financial burden to my parents.

So I lived in this world of gloom for 20 years. I finished high school, graduated from college, and entered the work world, struggling to stay alive, to stay involved, and to have some sort of happiness. I found it by involving my self as a recreation center worker. I was able to lose myself in my work, playing with boys and girls on the playground and in sports.

Still I was moody and hard to get along with. I was irritable and felt like a boiling cauldron. The least things could set me off. I had that typical "chip on my shoulder." I truly had a "bad attitude."

Eventually I earned a master's degree and went to work in an agency that had a psychiatrist on staff. He called me aside and talked to me about my depression. He prescribed my first anti-depressant medications. It took the edge off the depression.

What was your initial and later long-term reaction to the diagnosis?

With the first psychiatrist at age 15, I was uncomfortable, as I said. But when I had that second talk 20 years later, I really felt relieved that someone actually understood what I was feeling and had reached out to me. I mean, he sought me out. That blew me away. He cared about me as a person. Over the years, I had three or four other psychiatrists, but I never had that kind of relationship again. These later ones treated me as a patient, not a person, a friend.

How is your disorder treated?

I have been the rounds with psychotropic medications. I have taken tricyclic antidepressants (Norpramin), atypical antidepressants (Wellbutrin, Effexor, and Trazodone) {sic}, selected serotonin reuptake inhibitors (Zoloft), and serotonin noradrenalin reuptake inhibitors (Cymbalta.) None has really worked except the Cymbalta. It keeps me off the edge but never takes me to sunshine, so to speak.

I have been in outpatient counseling with a psychologist—actually two of them, inpatient hospitalization twice, behavioral therapy, and group therapy. I have had courses on anger management and stress management. I have had seven different psychiatrists over the course of 60 years.

Did you have to make any dietary or life style changes in response to your illness?

I should have altered my eating habits. I eat for comfort. Food is one of my best therapies. But, I can't afford to eat healthy, especially now that I am on Social Security. Fresh fruits and vegetables are expensive. So I eat lots of beans, potatoes, rice, and pastas. I was never big on sweets except for pies. I don't eat desserts except for special occasions. Or when someone has coconut cream pie.

Shopping has also been a great depression reliever. But I don't have the money to shop for nice things or electronics. All my furniture is from the 1970s. When I did shop, I overspent and went into debt and struggled with debt, payments, and credit cards. So I no longer have credit cards. I finally have learned how to live within my means, provided I don't have a financial crisis. I manage to eat out one time a month. It's my reward for getting through the previous month. It is my pleasurable event. It is always dinner alone. And I haven't been to a movie, concert or theater in 13 years. I don't have television.

In order to make significant lifestyle changes, though—especially in physical exercise and activity, I need motivation and energy to make those changes. Depression suppresses motivation and energy. It's a complicated cycle. I struggle with how to interrupt that cycle. I need a buddy to come over and say "Let's go!"

What other medical conditions do you have?

Diabetes, high blood pressure, high cholesterol, and sleep apnea. I also have diabetic neuropathy in both feet and a bit in my fingers. I have a lot of trouble with my balance and fall 3 or 4 times a month. But I refuse to give in to a cane or walker.

The blood pressure and cholesterol are well controlled with medications. I struggle with diabetes and with the sleep apnea. Treatment for those conditions is very expensive to keep on top of it.

What do you mean?

I have been on several medications for the diabetes and the one I am taking now does not completely do the job. With that medication alone, my blood sugars are about 240 to 350. At one point the reading was over 600. The A1C runs about 8.5 but was as high as 13 until I was put on an injection medication. Victoza.

That was doing the job and my blood sugars were down below 150, even below 100 a time or two and I felt like I was getting it under control. Then I hit that damn Medicare gap and my co-pay went from $45 to $158. It does so every August. I can't afford that so I go 5 months without it.

To top it off, the insurance carrier for Medicare stopped paying for that particular medication and I had to start a new one. It was working, but insufficient time was available before I once again hit the Medigap. It is very disheartening. I get so angry. It is very stressful trying to manage my diabetes, what with the problems with food and the gaps in prescription coverage.

What do you mean by problems with food?

Because I have very limited income, just the Social Security check, I usually end the month with $5 to $10 dollars left over. Sometimes I get overdrawn at the bank. To stay within budget, I have to rely on the community food pantry. I know they have constraints on them, but the two food boxes each month contain mostly rice, pasta, breads and sweets, and sugar coated cereals. (see Appendix 4) I should eat none of those items. None of them.

Usually I get 5 or 6 cans of something. On more than one occasion I received three cans of cranberry sauce. I have nine cans of the stuff in my pantry.

I decline the sweets and the cereals, but I do take home the rice dinners, pasta meals, and potatoes— boxes of potatoes au gratin or three cheese, and such as that. So in order to eat, I eat what I get in the food boxes. That doesn't help with the weight or the blood sugars. But what can I do?

Tell me about the sleep apnea.

I have been on a c-pap since 1996. The machine I have now is good and has been servicing me for about 8 years. The struggle is with the mask and supplies. And the doctors. I have had six of them. Only the current one has ever scheduled me for a follow up visit.

So when the time comes to replace a mask, hose, pillows, or filters it is a real hassle to get an appointment. Usually I delay as long as I can. I tape the broken mask back together and use safety pins for the worn out Velcro strips. It is such a chore to get out and drive 50 miles one way to go to a supplier.

And the on-line suppliers don't accept Medicare. That means that I get a few months of good sleep before the mask breaks or the straps wear out. Then I struggle every night to get a good night of sleep.

Medicare will pay for three or four replacements a year. But the co-pay is incredibly high. I can't afford to replace the mask or other supplies.

I can tell the difference when I don't get good sleep. Just like I can tell the difference when I run out of my anti-depressant. Within 2 days I am crying like a baby.

Did you seek any type of emotional support?

I did. I have. Bad experiences each time. I have attended support groups and outpatient group therapy. Mostly those sessions seemed pointless and non-directed.

Usually, someone in the group would get angry— especially if I didn't feel comfortable exposing my deepest secrets yet, and he or she would start attacking me. What good is that? And the group leaders usually let that go on. Not even some help in responding to the attack.

So I shy away from support groups. I have also experienced situations in which something shared in the confidentiality of the group came back to me from the secretary of one of the group members.

I have also sought help from an assistant pastor at a church. You know, churches are supposed to be full of loving, caring, and helpful people. I would expect that especially from the pastors. So I talked with this pastor and she was going to get someone to help me. No one ever contacted me. I was told that (name withheld) "will contact you when they get back from vacation." Never did. The pastor never followed up to make sure the contact had been made. She had "done her part." She had contacted someone to stand along side me.

Does your depression have any impact on your family?

I have outlived my family. No one remains but me, except for nieces and nephews from whom I never hear. I don't even know where 5 of them live or if they are married and have children. I do have some contact with three but it is on a superficial level. I try to have meaningful engagement. But they don't seem to have time. They are all so busy. I understand that. So they go about their lives without any consideration of me. Much the way we were with our aunts and uncles.

I also have 3 first cousins and a handful of second cousins scattered around the country. I do have contact on social media with a couple of cousins in California—some 2500 miles away or in Iowa.

In the past, when family was still alive, there were problems within the family. My mother tried to understand, once she realized I was not exaggerating or making things up in my head. In the years before she died she was very supportive.

One of my brothers told our mother that I was just neurotic and there was nothing wrong with me. He had a doctorate and thought he was God's gift to the world. Yeah, we didn't get along at all. His comments fed into how my mother felt about hypochondria until I was hospitalized and she had a conversation with my psychiatrist.

Because of the family dynamics, and having been picked on by my two older brothers, and because my father was alcoholic, I never had a positive relationship with my family.

I hold resentment toward my deceased brothers. Two of them used to abuse me. And one of those sexually. And they used to borrow gas money from me when I was maybe 10 years old, but they never paid any of it back. My parents didn't require it of them, either. I learned some lessons about money through them, though.

What lessons did you learn?

Paying off debts and paying back borrowed money isn't important. Money is a convenience and it's ok to use and manipulate others through money. If you are in a position of power, you can do what you want regarding other people's money. You don't have to be accountable for loans.

How could others have been more helpful?

That's really hard to say. On the one hand, I wanted people in my life. On the other hand, I really didn't want to be bothered. And like most teenagers and young adults struggling for identity and independence, I didn't want to be controlled.

However, that being said, over the years I have sent out signals to others in direct conversation or on social media that I was not doing well and needed help. I even talked some about suicide over the years. No one ever commented. Not a word from anyone.

Oh, wait. One person told me to stop whining and grow up. That was really helpful, you know? So I no longer comment on my feelings, but my anger does show up on social media at times.

I remember once coming to a realization that I had a .32 caliber snub nose pistol in my mouth. I was that close. I gave the pistol to a friend and have never owned a gun since.

I guess what would really be helpful is for someone to come by to pick me up and take me to lunch or dinner, invite me to attend a theater production or symphony performance with them, or just ride out to the country and buy some apples or grapes.

I am not likely to do any of those activities on my own initiative. The motivation and the money are not there. But then again, I don't want them to think I am just a freeloader. I sense that sometimes.

Sometimes I get overwhelmed with housekeeping. Dishes pile up in the sink. I try to wash everything after every meal, but sometimes my back hurts so badly it is difficult to stand over the sink. So before long dirty dishes, pots and pans, and utensils clutter the sink and counters.

Sometimes it would be helpful for someone to come over and say you just go sit down while I (we) give your house a good cleaning. For me, that would not be embarrassing or intrusive. But people shy away from that either because they don't want to embarrass me, don't have the time to be bothered, don't think about it, or because they really aren't that interested in what's going on in my life.

I know people are busy with their own lives and everyone has troubles of their own. Their own struggles keep them focused inward. I understand that.

I am told I should get involved in some community service to forget about my own problems. Well, my problems are with me every day and won't be forgotten.

But then, I get the point about getting involved in something beyond myself. I am willing to do that. So someone can come by, pick me up and take me to a community service agency and help me get started. Take action to support my desire to help others.

How are you doing at the present time?

I'm actually doing fairly well as far as the depression goes. The latest combination of Cymbalta and Welbutrin works well. I have feelings and moods that I don't remember having since before I was a teenager. Or rather, I am absent a lifetime of sadness, anxiety, despair, hopelessness—all that depression stuff is gone for now. It has taken 60 years to find the right combination.

What advice would you have for anyone living with depression?

Be prepared for a life long struggle. Be prepared to struggle alone. Be grateful for whatever help you get along the way. Come to a clear understanding of your depression and seek professional help as early as you can. And to quote the late British Prime Minister Winston

Churchill in a commencement address to graduating students, "Never give up. Never give up. Never give up."

SUMMARY

The interview with James demonstrates the thinking, behavior, mood, and attitude of one with a depressive disorder. Candid responses provide the opportunity to get inside the head of one person— and only that one person. The interview reveals some distorted thinking by James about his depression and his life circumstances. Interviews such as the one with James reveal additional insights about depressive disorders.

REVIEW QUESTIONS
(written or discussion)

1. How have these case scenarios helped you in your understanding of depression?

2. In what ways would you say that "James" has faulty interpretations about his depression and about the circumstances in which he finds himself?

3. What insights did you gain about James from the interview?

4. What more would you like to ask James about his life and about his depression?

5. In what ways do you think James is exaggerating his condition?

6. What is your overall impression of James?

7. Is James realistic in his expectations of others supporting him? Explain.

8. Identify any strength you see in James in coping with his life, his illnesses and his depression.

CLASS DISCUSSION

Discuss what you have learned about depression through the interview with James.

NOTES

9

Treatment Options: Medications

Now that a substantive understanding of depression has developed, we turn to treatment options. Treatment has come a long, long way over the past 75 years or so. The days of the diagnosis of "melancholia" are gone.

Except in some rare situations, electro-convulsive (shock) treatment does not frequently occur. When it does happen, advances in muscle relaxing medications have made it less likely that a person experiences adverse affects. Treatments that are more effective have reduced the use of electro-convulsive therapy that shot bursts of electrical impulses down the nerve fibers with force.

Some of the adverse effects of shock treatment were that it caused seizures and memory loss. Although effective, many considered it as "a last resort," which is not the case at all. It may be effective in some situations where the severely depressed patient is delusional or suicidal. However, severe depression may respond well to psychotropic medications and psychotherapy.

PSYCHOPHARMACOLOGY

Medications and pharmaceutical companies have taken a lot of criticism over recent years. Many people are critical of physicians and psychiatrists who they think over prescribe medications. Behaviorists claim that depression lessens or resolves by behavior modification without the use of drugs.

While it is true that abuse of prescribed medications can occur, over prescribing of certain medications may not be entirely the responsibility of the prescribing physician. In the case of medications for treating depression, physicians must rely not only on the physical appearance of the patient but also on self-reports of the patient herself. Inaccurate or incomplete self-reporting misguides the physician in some cases.

Once again, we must stress the importance of proper reporting of the appearance, behaviors and conversations of the patient. Considerable help is available to treat persistent depressive disorder, major depressive disorder, and other related conditions through medication provided the physician or psychiatrist has full disclosure of what is happening with the patient.

DIFFICULTY IN PRESCRIBING

At one time, only a few medicines were available in treating depression. Although knowing about neurotransmitters and their function, we did not have the expertise to determine which of the neurotransmitters were deficient in the synapses within the nerve system. A more general approach to medication was the result.

Although pharmaceutical companies designed medications in the 1960s and 1970s to correct deficiencies in norepinephrine and serotonin, physicians did not know which medication would be most effective.

A significant amount of trials was required to determine finally the most effective medication to prescribe. Sometimes, patients became discouraged because their medications did not seem to be working.

TYPES OF ANTIDEPRESSANTS

The list of antidepressants has grown considerably since the first ones developed in the late 1940s and early 1950s. We now look at four types or classes of these medications. (Appendix 5) We begin with the earliest ones and then on to current ones.

MONOAMINE OXIDASE INHIBITORS (MAOIs)

MAOIs were the first antidepressants to be developed. They fell out of favor because of concerns about interactions with certain foods and numerous drug interactions. Using MAOIs requires a strict diet because of dangerous (even deadly) interactions with certain foods such as some cheeses, pickles and wines and some medications including birth control pills, decongestants and certain herbal supplements.

MAOIs elevate the levels of norepinephrine, serotonin, and dopamine by inhibiting an enzyme called monoamine oxidase, which breaks down norepinephrine, serotonin, and dopamine. When monoamine oxidase is inhibited, norepinephrine, serotonin, and dopamine are not broken down, increasing the concentration of these three neurotransmitters in the brain. Parkinson's disease patients sometimes use them for treatment of that disorder.

TRICYCLIC MEDICATIONS

These antidepressants—such as imipramine (Tofranil), nortriptyline (Pamelor), (Surmontil), desipramine (Norpramin) and protriptyline (Vivactil), work by increasing the concentrations of two mood-altering chemicals norepinephrine and serotonin in the brain. Scientists are not sure how tricyclics work. Biochemical and medical personnel think tricyclic medications work to increase neurotransmitter levels by preventing nerve endings—called synapses, from drawing these chemicals back into their tissues, which is normally how the body reduces their concentrations. Figure 2 depicted neurotransmitters and the synapse.

SIDE EFFECTS

Another issue with the earlier medications, the trycyclics, was potential for severe side effects. Some of the common side effects include:

- Dry mouth
- Blurred vision
- Sweating
- Dizziness or lightheadedness
- Drowsiness
- Restlessness
- Racing heartbeat
- Increased sweating
- Urinary retention
- Constipation
- Tremor

- Increased appetite
- Weight gain
- Low sex drive
- Difficulty achieving an erection, and other sexual difficulties
- Low blood pressure when rising to a stand
- Confusion in the elderly

Tricyclic medications may also increase the potential and risk in some people for suicide. Physicians seldom prescribe tricyclic medications now unless the more recent medications, such as the selective serotonin reuptake inhibitors (SSRIs), provide poor results.

REUPTAKE INHIBITORS

Reuptake inhibitors are just what the words indicate. They function to prevent the reuptake of neurotransmitters within the synapse when the neurons are not replenishing them. Refer once again to Figure 2 for a diagram of the nerve endings, synapse, and hormone neurotransmitters. The following list includes the neurotransmitter reuptake inhibitors.

Selective serotonin reuptake inhibitors

These medications are the first choice of most physicians and psychiatrists in the treatment of depressive disorders. These medications tend to have fewer side effects than others do. This group of medications works to inhibit the reuptake of serotonin in the synapses.

Most of the body's serotonin is located in the gastrointestinal tract. The body must produce serotonin used inside the brain within the brain itself. Biochemists and physicians think that serotonin affects mood, social behavior, appetite, digestion, sleep, memory and sexual desire and function. Selective serotonin reuptake inhibitors (SSRIs) include fluoxetine (Prozac), paroxetine (Paxil, Pexeva), sertraline (Zoloft), citalopram (Celexa) and escitalopram (Lexapro).

Serotonin-norepinephrine reuptake inhibitors (SNRIs)

On the other hand, norepinephrine is a hormone that energizes the body and causes activity and movement. Sometimes known as the stress hormone, it triggers the body's "fight-flight" function. Examples of SNRIs include duloxetine (Cymbalta), venlafaxine (Effexor XR), desvenlafaxine (Pristiq, Khedezla) and levomilnacipran (Fetzima). SNRIs work to inhibit both serotonin and norepinephrine.

Norepinephrine-dopamine reuptake inhibitors (NDRIs)

Next, we come to an inhibitor in the reuptake of the neurotransmitter dopamine as well as norepinephrine. Dopamine is a neurotransmitter hormone located deep in the brain. It assists in the start of movement. Its absence or insufficiency in the brain is a contributor to Parkinson's disease.

Dopamine affects a person's emotions and the sensations of pleasure and pain. Because of this function, dopamine has a relationship to reward and punishment behaviors. Bupropion (Wellbutrin, Aplenzin, and Forfivo XL) falls into this category. It's one of the few antidepressants not frequently associated with sexual side effects.

Figure 6 shows the neurotransmitters dopamine, norepinephrine, and serotonin with their action and their contribution to a person's mood.

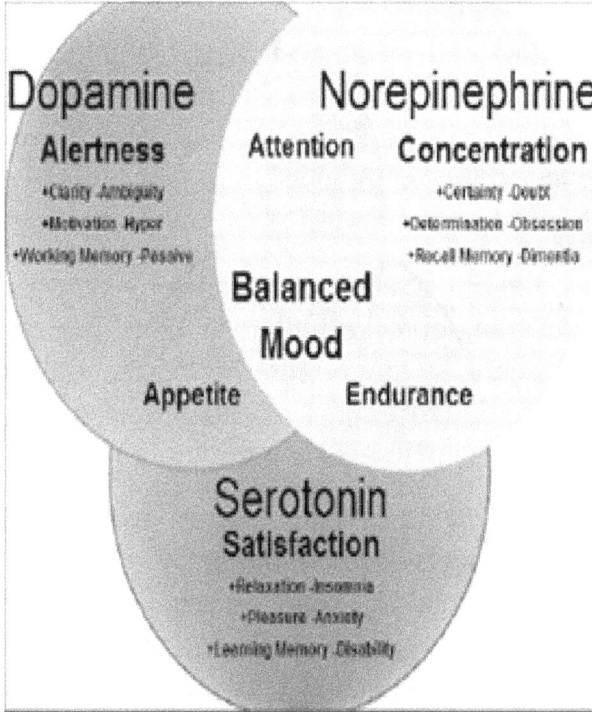

Figure 6: Neurotransmitters, their actions, and effect on mood

ATYPICAL ANTIDEPRESSANTS

Atypical antidepressants medications do not fit into any other antidepressant categories. Trazodone and mirtazapine (Remeron) are sedating medications usually taken in the evening. Newer medications include vortioxetine (Brintellix) and vilazodone (Viibryd). Vilazodone may have a low risk of sexual side effects.

Physicians use trazodone in some cases for treatment of sleep apnea.

RISK CONSIDERATIONS

Watch closely anyone taking an antidepressant for worsening depression or unusual behavior, especially when first beginning a new medication or with a change in dosage. If someone has suicidal thoughts when taking an antidepressant, contact the physician or a hospital emergency room immediately. Keep in mind that antidepressants are more likely to reduce suicide risk over time by improving mood.

Another consideration is short-term increased fear or anxiety. Often depressed mood is the body's response to fear or anxiety. As the depression lifts, conditions that it suppressed may reoccur. This situation also needs careful monitoring in the short term.

Because these conditions arise, and in order to make significant gains in treatment, medications may be more effective if combined with counseling or psychotherapy. As the medications restore the body and the brain, any conditions in lifestyle, emotional, or psychological areas may need consideration. Mental health professionals such as psychiatrists, psychologists, psychological examiners, licensed clinical social workers, psychiatric nurses, and family life counselors provide these services in private practice or through an agency.

SUMMARY

Treatment has come a long, long way over the past 75 years or so. Treatments that are more effective have reduced the use of electro-convulsive therapy and some of the earliest psychotropic medications. Seldom used today, Monoamine oxidase inhibitors (MAOI) and tricyclic antidepressants, gave way to new classes of medications that seem more effective.

Behaviorists claim that behavior modification without the use of drugs can lessen or resolve depression. However, medications remain a standard course of treatment by physicians and psychiatrists. Behavioral therapies usually occur in hospital or treatment centers in which staff controls the environment.

We now look to four types or classes of these medications for treating depression. Monoamine oxidizer inhibitors (MOAIs) and tricyclic antidepressants, the first two classes of these medications, have certain use constraints or side effects that preclude their use as a first choice in treatment of depression. Reuptake inhibitors and atypical antidepressants seem to have the most effectiveness in treating of depressive disorders. Some antidepressant medications may have associated risk factors.

These medications appear to inhibit the reuptake of hormones such as serotonin, norepinephrine, and dopamine until the body develops ability to restore levels of these hormones to proper levels for functioning. Because some environmental stressors contribute to depression in some people, physicians and psychiatrists often recommend other therapeutic interventions such as psychotherapy simultaneous with the use of medications.

REVIEW QUESTIONS

(written or discussion)

1. What are four classes of medications used in the treatment of depression?

2. T F Risk factors need not be considered when taking antidepressants because they are not addictive in nature.

3. T F Suicidal thoughts sometimes occur as a person's depression lifts.

4. T F Monoamine oxidase inhibitors have dietary risk factors.

5. Antidepressants appear to prevent the reuptake of _____ in the synapse.

6. Name three hormones frequently associated with depression.

7. T F Antidepressant medications may be used is some cases in treatment of other disorders such as Parkinson's disease or sleep apnea.

8. T F Psychotherapy may be recommended with use of antidepressant medications.

CLASS DISCUSSION

How do antidepressants work in the treatment of depressive disorders? What, if any, are the risk factors associated with use of antidepressants? Include all previous chapters in your discussion.

10

Psychotherapy And Counseling

Talk therapy. Psychoanalysis. The psychiatrist's couch. These are some of the common images of psychotherapy and counseling.

Psychotherapy is a general term for treating depression by talking about the patient's condition and related issues with a mental health provider. Psychotherapy refers to talk therapy or psychological therapy. This type of therapy involves regular interaction between a trained clinician and a patient (or in some instances, a group of patients.)

Psychotherapists have training in a variety of techniques to help patients to recover from mental illness, resolve personal issues, and create desired changes in their lives. Just as no two people suffer the exact same way with depression, no universal treatment that cures depression exists. What works for one person might not work for another. The best way to treat depression is to become as informed as possible about the patient's circumstances and treatment options, and then tailor them to meet client needs.

Let us once again reinforce the importance of accurate and comprehensive assessments. These assessments will provide significant and other information. The treatment team will find all the comprehensive assessments very useful in developing a personalized treatment plan and not one that is actually a cookie cutter plan under the guise of an "individual" treatment plan.

Different types of psychotherapy can be effective for depression – such as cognitive behavioral therapy or interpersonal therapy. The mental health provider also may recommend other therapies. Psychotherapy can help adjust to a crisis or other current difficulty and Identify negative thoughts, beliefs and behaviors and replace them with healthy, positive ones. Exploring relationships and experiences, and developing positive interactions with others can occur in various talk therapies.

Finding better ways to cope and solve problems and Identify issues that contribute to depression and change behaviors that make it worse are benefits of talk therapy. Working as or with a professional counselor helps to regain a sense of satisfaction and control in one's life and help ease depression symptoms, such as hopelessness and anger. One can learn to set realistic goals for life and develop the ability to tolerate and accept distress using healthier behaviors.

COMMON TYPES OF PSYCHOTHERAPY

The most common types of psychotherapy used in the treatment of depression are varied and range from cognitive therapies to behavioral treatments. They occur in several formats including individual, group, couples, and family therapy sessions. The following overviews are helpful in understanding how treatment occurs and what the expectations from such are.

Cognitive Therapy

Based on the idea that thoughts affect and control our behavior, cognitive therapy focuses on the patient thinking patterns. Cognitive therapy seeks to condition the brain to replace negative though patterns with positive ones. Going back to Figure 4, cognitive therapy seeks to change those memory tapes and replace them with new, positive thoughts.

Cognitive therapy helps to identify common patterns of negative thinking. Clinicians call this negative thinking cognitive distortion. This type of psychotherapy may require anti-depressant medications to improve the patient's cognitive functioning along with the cognitive therapy.

Behavioral Therapy

Behavioral therapy focuses on changing undesired behaviors, using principles of classical and operant conditioning in order to reinforce wanted behaviors while eliminating unwanted behaviors. Behavior therapy considers that behavior is what matters, meaning how one behaves overrides how one thinks. Thinking will change based on changed behaviors.

The difficulty with behavioral therapies is in control of the social and psychological environment. Elimination of negative behaviors requires positive reinforcement. Consequences apply to negative behavior.

Another consideration in applying behavioral therapy to depression is the notion that some depressions are genetic in nature. Would behavioral therapy be able to override this condition and change a person's mood, affect, and cognition? The answer seems undecided, although strict behavioralists say yes.

Cognitive Behavioral Therapy

While behavioral therapy is effective in the treatment of depression, its primary use is with behavioral disorders. Clinicians use it frequently in treatment of children and adolescents and certain chronic mental illnesses.

Cognitive therapy and behavioral therapy work well in combination with each other. Treatment for depression and anxiety disorders often occur using cognitive behavioral therapy.

Dialectical Behavioral Therapy

Dialectical behavioral therapy is an extension of cognitive behavioral therapy based on the philosophical concept of dialectics. Dialectics holds that everything composes as opposites and that change occurs when one opposing force is stronger than the other is. This type of psychotherapy is a foundation of Kurt Lewin's Field of Forces Analysis but incorporates some mindfully aware notions of Buddhist tradition.

Kurt Lewin's Field of Forces Analysis

Lewin's force field analysis identifies opposing forces that control behaviors and thinking. These forces are driving forces and restraining forces interacting to cause behaviors. The driving forces, of course, drive a certain behavior while the restraining forces counter those driving forces. Where more or stronger driving forces exist, the identified trouble behavior occurs and may increase.

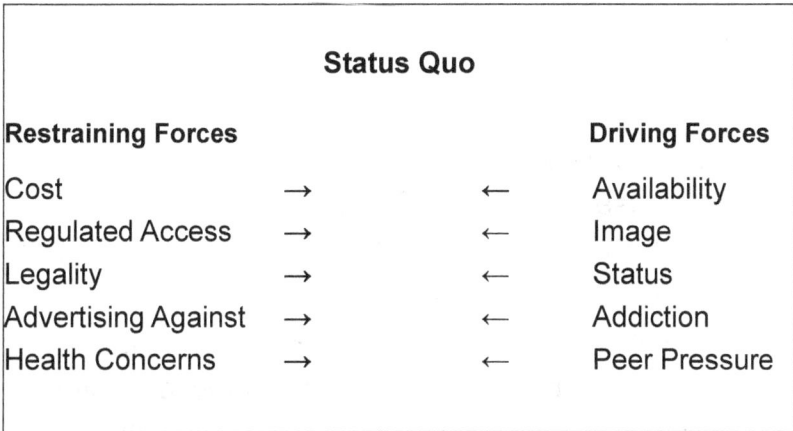

Status Quo		
Restraining Forces		**Driving Forces**
Cost	→ ←	Availability
Regulated Access	→ ←	Image
Legality	→ ←	Status
Advertising Against	→ ←	Addiction
Health Concerns	→ ←	Peer Pressure

Figure 7: Field of Forces Analysis Example

Figure 7 demonstrates the force field analysis of smoking cigarettes. Understand that the analysis can apply to an individual, a community, or a society. The same principle applies to all circumstances.

The forces that drive up the smoking of cigarettes in this example include availability, addiction, habit, advertising, peer pressure, and anxiety. Of course, this example is simplistic for the purposes of teaching about the concept.

The restraining forces include cost, legal age, anti-smoking campaign, societal considerations, and fear of lung cancer. To reduce the smoking behavior the restraining forces must be strengthened or new restraints added. One approach could include reducing the strength of the driving forces, such as changing peers.

Interpersonal Therapy

Interpersonal therapy focuses on past and present social roles and interpersonal interactions. Through therapeutic intervention, the therapist generally chooses one or two areas of concern in the patient's current life to focus on.

Psychodynamic Therapy

Psychodynamic therapy assumes that unresolved conflicts cause depression. These conflicts may have occurred in childhood or adolescents. The patient may be unaware of the existence of these conflicts.

Psychodynamic therapy treatment seeks to make the patient or client more aware of their emotions, often contradictory in nature and of how these emotions affect feeling, behavior, and cognition. Psychodynamic therapy seeks to assist the patient or client in how to bear these feelings and put them into a more useful viewpoint perspective. This type of therapy developed from psychoanalysis.

PSYCHOANALYSIS

Psychoanalysis is the classic form of psychological therapy introduced by Sigmund Freud. Psychoanalytic therapy is an in-depth talk therapy that seeks to bring unconscious or deeply buried thoughts and feelings to the conscious mind so that any or all repressed experiences and emotions, often stemming from childhood, can be brought to the surface and examined. Working together, the therapist and client look at how these repressed early memories have affected the client's thinking, behavior, moods, and relationships in adulthood.

Psychoanalysis takes months or even years to accomplish its goals. Because of this fact, psychoanalysis is very expensive in most situations. Many years of training are required for a therapist to become adept in the techniques of psychoanalysis.

SUMMARY

Psychotherapy is a general term for treating depression by talking about the patient's condition and related issues with a mental health provider. Psychotherapy refers to talk therapy or psychological therapy. This type of therapy involves regular interaction between a trained clinician and a patient (or in some instances, a group of patients.)

No universal treatment that cures depression exists. Accurate and comprehensive assessments provide significant information for the clinical treatment team in developing a comprehensive treatment plan. Different types of psychotherapy can be effective for depression.

Psychotherapy can help adjust to a crisis or other current difficulty and Identify negative thoughts, beliefs and behaviors and replace them with healthy, positive ones. Finding better ways to cope and solve problems and Identify issues that contribute to depression and change behaviors that make it worse are benefits of talk therapy. Setting realistic goals for life and develop the ability to tolerate and accept distress using healthier behaviors can result from psychotherapy.

The most common types of psychotherapy used in the treatment of depression are varied and range from cognitive therapies to behavioral treatments. They occur in several formats including individual, group, couples, and family therapy sessions. These treatment options address two of the domains of development and function mentioned in Chapter 1.

Cognitive therapies focus on patient thinking patterns. Right thinking causes right behaviors. Behavioral therapies focus on changing undesired behaviors, using principles of classical and operant conditioning in order to reinforce wanted behaviors while eliminating unwanted behaviors. Right behaviors cause right thinking.

REVIEW QUESTIONS

(written or discussion)

1. T F Psychoanalysis is a short duration and inexpensive form of psychotherapy.

2. T F Psychotherapy refers to talk therapy or psychological therapy.

3. Behavioral therapies focus on changing undesired behaviors.

4. Behavior therapy uses _____ and

   _____ _____.

5. Cognitive therapies focus on patient's

   _____.

6. The most common forms of psychotherapy range from _____ to _____.

7. T F No universal treatment that cures depression
   exists.

8. T Different types of psychotherapy can be
   effective for depression.

CLASS DISCUSSION

Break into smaller groups and choose a behavior
for modification. Using the Field of Forces analysis,
identify possible driving and restraining forces. How could
the negative forces (can be either driving or restraining
forces) be altered?

NOTES

11

Other Treatment Options

Briefly, the following list of additional options provides insight into locations and newer forms of treatment. We also revisit Electro-Convulsive Therapy (ECT) as a treatment option. We start with locations as treatment setting options.

WHERE TREATMENT CAN OCCUR

The treatment setting may vary. Cost is not the only consideration. Sometimes the setting in which a patient is treated has beneficial results. These options range from private sessions in an outpatient clinic or private practice office setting to total inpatient care in a hospital.

Hospital and Residential Treatment

In some people, depression is so severe that the patient needs a hospital stay. This may be necessary if one cannot care for oneself properly or when one is in immediate danger of harming oneself or someone else. Psychiatric treatment at a hospital can help keep the patient calm and safe until mood improves and risks abate. In today's financial market place, insurance companies are reluctant to pay for hospital stays that do not have a risk of harming oneself or someone else.

In an inpatient setting, the depressed person may be involved with a psychiatrist who heads a treatment team and who prescribes and monitors medications. The team most likely includes a psychologist or a psychological (or psych) examiner, a licensed clinical social worker, a nutritionist, a hospital pharmacist, a physical therapist, an activity therapist, and a psychiatric nurse. This team approach provides for testing and psychotherapy, nutritional and diet plans, exercise and body strengthening, discharge planning, and a variety of classes to help with understanding the patient's condition and treatment plan.

Partial Hospitalization / Day Treatment

Partial hospitalization or day treatment programs also may help some people. These programs provide the outpatient support and counseling needed to get symptoms under control. Such options divert many people from inpatient care, allowing them to stay at home. They also keep the depressed individual in daily contact with the issues and conditions affecting the person, causing a face-to-face real time experience and treatment.

Outpatient Offices and Clinics

Most people receive support and treatment in outpatient clinics or private practice offices. Such settings provide regular, on-going counseling and psychotherapy sessions or medication reviews by the various clinicians treating the individual. These settings are by far the least expensive ones for treatment options.

Often, mental health agencies offer after care support groups. A professional clinician or a peer leads these groups. Support groups allow individuals the opportunity to share their feelings and their experiences with people in similar circumstances. Occurring on a regular and frequent basis enables a person with depression to continue to gain insights, to ventilate feelings, and to help other members of the group.

OTHER THERAPY OPTIONS

Let us look now at four addition treatment options that sometimes become appropriate. One is the earliest treatment for depression, electroconvulsive therapy. One, aversion therapy, finds its usefulness with chemical dependency and sexual addiction treatment settings. One seems sometimes successful in treatment of another disorder. The fourth one has a relatively new appearance on the scene.

Electroconvulsive Therapy

Electroconvulsive therapy (ECT) has a blemished reputation but a well-established efficacy in severe depression. It is one form of neuromodulation considered. As noted earlier, new procedures have eased some of the problems with ECT. Some memory loss still may occur with this procedure.

Aversion Therapy

Aversion therapy is a type of behavior therapy in which an aversive (causing a strong feeling of dislike or disgust) stimulus is coupled with an undesirable behavior in order to reduce or eliminate that behavior. Verbal aversion therapy, also known as covert sensitization, is a specific type of aversion therapy that does not involve the use of physical or "overt" stimuli — such as electrical shocks or nausea-inducing medications, to form an association between the undesirable behavior and an unpleasant effect or consequence. Aversion therapy is a behavioral treatment intervention based on the principles of classical conditioning and behavioral psychology. Sometimes people refer to aversion therapy as conversion therapy or reparative therapy.

Transcranial magnetic stimulation (TMS)

Transcranial magnetic stimulation (TMS) may be an option for those who have not responded to antidepressants. During TMS, the patient sits in a reclining chair, awake, with a treatment coil placed against one's scalp. The coil sends brief magnetic pulses to stimulate nerve cells in the brain that are involved in mood regulation and depression. Typically, patients have five treatments each week for up to six weeks.

Transcranial and Vagus Nerve Stimulation

The Federal Drug Administration (FDA) approves repetitive transcranial magnetic stimulation and vagus nerve stimulation for treating depression. Vagus nerve stimulation is a known procedure in treatment for epilepsy. The vagus nerve is responsible for some involuntary behavior such as regulating heartbeat and digestion.

SUMMARY

Treatment setting may vary. Cost is not the only consideration. Sometimes the setting in which a patient is treated has beneficial results.

For some, depression is so severe that the patient needs a hospital stay. Close monitoring of medications for these individuals requires it. For others, this may be necessary if one cannot care for oneself properly. Risk of suicide or harm to others also requires hospitalization.

Day treatment or partial hospitalization services provide care during full day or part of the day care and activities for individuals with depression. Profession led or peer led outpatient support groups offer continuing after care activities and sharing of experiences. They allow patients to support each other in coping with their disorders.

The most common setting for the treatment of depressive disorders is the outpatient office setting. Clinicians in private practice or in agencies offer weekly, or sometimes only periodic, counseling or psychotherapy. Physicians and psychiatrists use outpatient settings to monitor and adjust patient use of medications.

The Federal Drug Administration has approved vagus nerve stimulation, a known procedure in treatment for epilepsy, as a treatment for depression. Transcranial magnetic stimulation (TMS) may be an option for those who have not responded to antidepressants.

REVIEW QUESTIONS

(written or discussion)

1. When is hospitalization for depression necessary?
2. How does a peer support group help the individual experiencing depression?
3. What is the most common setting for treatment for depression?
4. What is the least restrictive setting for treatment of depression?
5. Identify the earliest form of treatment for depression.
6. Who leads a peer support group? How are they qualified to lead the group?
7. Vagus nerve stimulation is a known treatment for _____ as well as depression.

CLASS DISCUSSION

Discuss the pros and cons of a team approach in the treatment of depression. What factors need consideration? How do various members contribute to quality patient care? What is the most important thing to consider in treating a person with a depressive disorder?

12

Trends And Research

The treatment for depression has come under scrutiny in the past several years. Psychologists and others debunk the use of medications as an effective treatment for depression, holding that the various forms of behavioral therapies are better approaches.

Critics of use of medications, most of whom have never treated a patient for depression, have inundated the various media with allegations that medications – which have helped patients for decades, are no better than placebos.

Several major pharmaceutical companies have scaled down or disengaged their research into new anti-depressant medications. Treatment resistant depression appears to be on the up rise with no new mechanisms of action coming along. New kinds of approaches and research seem the current trend in treatment and resolution of depressive disorders.

NEW APPROACHES

New approaches explore an array for consideration. Let us look at these following models:

Genetics and the Environment

For decades clinicians thought that "endogenous" depression resulted from genetic influences while "exogenous" depression was the result of some environmental factor. Currently researchers are looking at how environmental influences interact with the genetic structure of the individual. This research would suggest that having a genetic risk for depression might not actually be causal for the disorder without certain environmental influences.

Chemical Imbalance and Inflammatory Processes

Some evidence is showing that inflammation may be behind depression. Studies have shown that cytokines and interleukins increase during a depressive episode and decrease as the depression abates.

Neurotransmitters, Neuroplasticity, and Neurotropic Factors

Current medication treatment for depression appears designed to increase or maintain the levels of neurotransmitters in the brain. New research reveals that depression is associated with a significant drop in neurotropic factors such as brain derived neurotropic factor (BDNF) or fibroblast growth factor with a concomitant decline in hippocampal neurogenesis. Neurotrophins are important regulators for survival, differentiation, and maintenance of nerve cells. They are small proteins that secrete into the nervous system to help keep nerve cells alive.

Serotonin, Norepinephrine, Dopamine, and Glutamate

Over the past few years, glutamate pathways and the glutamate N-methyl-D-aspartate (NMDA) receptor have become an important focus in the link between neurobiology and the occurrence of depression. This link between the strong therapeutic effects of antagonizing the NMDA receptor in depression and the increase in BDNF and neuroplasticity seems to have emerged as a fresh representation of depression.

Pills or Intravenous Infusions

Some studies show that a single infusion of the NMDA receptor antagonist ketamine produces a very vigorous response, including full remission, in treatment–resistant unipolar or bipolar depression within 1 to 2 hours. The mechanism of action seems caused by a surge of BDNF and immediate neuroplastic changes following NMDA receptor blockade. This abrupt reversal of severe depression occurred in limited studies. These limited studies show promise for a larger population. Research continues.

Pharmacology and Neuromodulation

Ingested medications disseminate into all the body's organs and not just the brain. Because of this action, unwanted side effects to the medications can occur. Neuromodulation, electric and magnetic treatment forms, stimulate specific parts of the brain.

The HPA Axis

The Hypothalamic Pituitary Adrenal (HPA) axis is a commonly observed neuroendocrine abnormality in patients suffering from major depressive disorder (MDD). Altered cortisol secretion appears in as many as 80% of these depressed patients. Research seeks better to understand the molecular mechanisms, which underlie the alteration of the HPA axis responsiveness in depressive illness.

Agents that intervene with the mechanisms involved in (dys)regulation of cortisol synthesis and release are under investigation as possible therapeutic agents. Studies continue in the variant to typical treatment options for depression.

Clearly biomedical science has come far in the understanding of the causes of depression from the notions of melancholia and neurotic behavior. Breakthroughs are expected.

RESULTANT NEW PRACTICES

The resulting progress made in the understanding the causes of and treatment for depression has produced some interesting and possibly significant gains. Based on some recent research, several approved new approaches are now in use. Let us look at some of these.

Other forms of neuromodulation, such as cranial electrical stimulation, epidural cortical stimulation, focused ultrasound, low field magnetic stimulation, magnetic seizure therapy, near infrared light therapy, and transcranial direct current stimulation still are in development. Deep brain stimulation (DBS) shows in several recent studies to reverse TRD especially when stimulating the subgenual anterior cingulated region. In the future, DBS may become as commonly used in depression as it currently is in Parkinson's disease.

BRAIN IMAGING

Studies out of Johns Hopkins University medical center show what some call amazing or staggering results from brain imaging of people with unremitting, depression. Renowned neurologist Helen S. Mayberg, M.D. stated that depression first is a brain disease. Brain-imagining technologies allow scientists to look at the regional patterns of brain activity and determine how the specific circuits of the brain differ in persons who are depressed versus "normal," non-depressed people.[9]

Pharmacologists and psychiatrists have consistently concentrated mostly with the overall chemistry in the brain—the imbalances of neurotransmitters, without looking into the abnormalities in different regions of the brain and the activities in those problem spots that may be contributing to stubborn depression. Neurologists like Mayberg use brain-mapping techniques to discover what occurs inside the brain and how those functions connect to mood.

The neurological perspective—focusing on specific brain circuits, differs from, but is complementary to, the biochemical approach of drug therapy, which affects the action of cells throughout the entire brain, in whatever region they are located. An entirely new approach for developing targeted treatments is now foreseeable.

---

9   Helen Mayberg, MD, The Johns Hopkins Depression & Anxiety Bulletins.

SUMMARY

Psychologists and others debunk the use of medications as an effective treatment for depression, holding that the various forms of behavioral therapies are the better approaches. Treatment resistant depression appears to be on the up rise. New kinds of approaches and research seem the current trend in treatment and resolution of depressive disorders.

Currently researchers are looking at how environmental influences interact with the genetic structure of the individual. Areas of current research include 1) genetics and the environment, 2) chemical imbalance and inflammatory processes, 3) neurotransmitters, neuroplasticity, and neurotropic factors, 4) hormones and esters such as serotonin, norepinephrine, dopamine, and glutamate, 5) pills or intravenous infusions, and 6) pharmacology and neuromodulation. The Hypothalamic Pituitary Adrenal (HPA) axis is a commonly observed neuroendocrine abnormality in patients suffering from major depressive disorder (MDD).

Neuromodulation, electric and magnetic treatment forms, stimulate specific parts of the brain. Cranial electrical stimulation, epidural cortical stimulation, focused ultrasound, low field magnetic stimulation, magnetic seizure therapy, near infrared light therapy, and transcranial direct current stimulation remain in development. Deep brain stimulation and brain scanning techniques may provide new approaches. The neurological perspective—focusing on specific brain circuits, differs from, but is complementary to, the biochemical approach of drug therapy, which affects the action of cells throughout the entire brain, in whatever region they are located.

REVIEW QUESTIONS
(written or discussion)

1. T F Many behavioralists reject the use of medications for treatment of depression.

2. T F Treatment resistant depression is decreasing with newer forms of treatment.

3. Researchers are now exploring how environmental influences interact with _____ of the individual.

4. Name four areas of research occurring in the treatment of depressive disorders.

5. What is neuromodulation?

6. The _____ perspective focuses on specific brain circuits.

CLASS DISCUSSION

How effective are current practices in the treatment of depressive disorders? What are some of the drawbacks? What do you think is the future for neuro-pharmacology versus some of the newer approaches not involving medication?

NOTES

13

Resources And Support

For someone experiencing depression, it is important to know that this individual is not alone and that the condition is treatable. Here is a list of depression organizations, articles, and websites for more information and support.

Organizations

- National Alliance on Mental Illness: 1-800-950-NAMI (1-800-950-6264) //www.nami.org
- Anxiety and Depression Association of America: 1-240-485-1001, //www.adaa.org
- National Institute of Mental Health:
- 1-866-615-6464,//www. nimh.gov
- Centers for Disease Control and Prevention: Division of Mental Health, 1-800-CDC-INFO (1-800-232-4636) //www.cdc.gov/mentalhealth
- American Psychological Association:
- 1-800-374-2721, //www.apa.org
- American Psychiatric Association: 1-703-907-7300, //www.psychiatry.org
- Mental Health America (formerly the Mental Health Association) https://www.cchrint.org/issues/psycho-pharmaceutical-front-groups/mha/

- <u>National Institute of Mental Health - NIH</u> *https:// www.nimh.nih.gov/*
- Your State Department of Mental Health or Mental Hygiene
- Your local Community Mental Health Center

Financial Assistance

- Partnership for Prescription Assistance: //www/ pparx.org
- NeedyMeds: 1-800-503- 6897 //www.needymeds. org
- Together Rx Access //www.togetherrxaccess.com
- Social Security Administration //www.ssa.gov
- CareForYourMind.org

Coping, Advocacy, and Support

- Anxiety and Depression Association of America: https://adaa.org/support Groups
- American Foundation for Suicide Prevention: 1-800-273-TALK (1-800-273-8255), //afsp.org
- Depression and Bipolar Support Alliance: 1-800-826-3632, //www.dbsalliance.org
- Families for Depression Awareness: 1-781-890-0220, //familyaware.org
- To Write Love On Her Arms: 1-800-273-TALK (1-800-273-8255), //twloha.com

One can also look for Psychiatrists, psychologists, and social workers in the local telephone directories. It is important for social workers, especially clinical social workers, to remember that many individuals suffering with depression have impaired cognitive processes. Because of this fact, these individuals may not be able personally to access these resources or to seek services from them.

Therefore, the role of the social worker is more than intake and referral or psychotherapy. It is for the clinical social worker more than just counsel and referral. *Social workers must be willing and available to their clients and patients to contact these resources and arrange services for the individuals in their caseload or practice.*

SUMMARY

Depression is treatable. Support is available from a number of local, state, and national organizations that provide information, financial assistance, and assistance for coping and advocacy. It is important to know that the depressed individual and the family are not alone.

However, many individuals suffering with depression have impaired cognitive processes. Because of this fact, these individuals may not be able personally to access these resources or to seek services from them. A referral to another agency or service is insufficient in many cases.

Therefore, the role of the social worker is more than intake and referral or psychotherapy. It is for the clinical social worker more than just counsel and referral. Social workers must be willing and available to their clients and patients to contact these resources and arrange services for the individuals in their caseload or practice.

Social workers must always retain their function as grass roots change agents. Too often social work roles in private practice and in mental health treatment facilities have lost that grass roots aspect of change agent. Social workers must be willing to make that telephone call to another agency, to advocate for their clients, and to be more than a therapist or a referral source.

Sometimes action is required.

REVIEW QUESTIONS
(written or discussion)

1. Name four organizations that provide information about depressive disorders.

2. Identify two organizations that may offer financial support for people with depression.

3. List three national organizations that provide assistance in advocacy, support, and coping for depressed individuals and their families.

CLASS DISCUSSION

Referral to agencies is an important role for social workers. Discuss the most effective ways of making referrals and seeking services for clients suffering with a depressive disorder. What is necessary in follow-up of a referral? What is the difference in follow-up and follow-through on referrals to other agencies and services? What is the role of the licensed clinical social worker whose primary function is providing counseling and psychotherapy in follow-through?

NOTES

14

Self-Help And Family Support

We cannot emphasize the importance of seeking professional help enough. Depression can be a life changing and a life-threatening condition if not properly treated in a timely and professional manner. Psychiatrists, psychologists, psychological examiners, licensed clinical social workers, and psychiatric nurses have expertise and years of training in the areas of mental health that provide the depressed individual with the best possible opportunity for recovery.

Too many friends of depressed individuals provide uninformed, inaccurate, and sometimes dangerous advice. Many of these friends (or in some instances family) advise against medications, propose organic cures, or just say the condition comes from a weakness of character. They regard use of medications as a sign of weakness in the individual.

"Be strong" is the mantra of these people. "You just need to resolve not to be depressed," as though depression is a choice. Depressed people should avoid these friends' advice and solutions.

Some people are reluctant to take anti-depressant medications because they do not want to be come dependent or addicted to them. Some who are vegetarians or vegans or who are strong advocates of organic and whole foods also reject the notion of medications for treatment of depression. This is incorrect thinking.

Some alternative medicines and herbal concoctions may have some minimal effect on relieving some of the symptoms of depression. However, because of the complexity of the depressive disorders—the various causes and possible treatment options, self-treatment with most alternative options may be unwise.

WHAT A DEPRESSED INDIVIDUAL CAN DO

This said, there exist several actions that the person suffering with a depressive disorder might do in addition to seeking professional help. The suggested items following are some of those steps to take.

Depression drains one's energy, hope, and motivation. Doing the essentials of life to feel better becomes difficult. Although overcoming depression is not quick or easy, it is far from impossible.

One cannot just will oneself to "snap out of it," but one does have more control than one realizes—even if the depression is severe and stubbornly persistent. The key is to start small and build from there. Feeling better takes time, but the depressed individual can get there by making positive choices each day.

Foundational Techniques

Have a mindfulness attitude, especially if one's depression is rooted in unresolved trauma or fed by obsessive, negative thoughts. Focus on how one's body feels as one moves—such as the sensation of one's feet hitting the ground, or the feeling of the wind on one's skin, or the rhythm of one's breathing.

Here are some foundational techniques for self-help for depression:

- **Mindfulness** – through breathing or engaging the 5 senses

- **Distraction** – Put the thoughts/feelings aside and come back to them when one are ready to deal with them

- **Positive Affirmations** – Have some affirmations written down repeat them to one's self daily. It has been said that it takes 7 positive affirmations to offset 1 negative one.

- **Sleep/Exercise/Diet** – All 3 aspects of our lifestyle can impact the way we think/feel.

- **Increasing Pleasurable Activities** – Engage in at least one pleasurable activity per day.

- **Focus** – acupuncture, guided imagery, yoga, meditation, breathing exercises, massage therapy

COPE WITH THE DEPRESSION

For starters, coping with depression is a Catch-22. Recovering from depression requires action, but taking action when one is depressed is not as easy as it sounds. Depression's nature is lack of energy, cognitive issues, withdrawal and social isolation, and lack of interest in former favorite activities.

However, as much as one is able, do things on a daily basis, starting slowly and simply and gradually building up these actions over several months. Do not expect magic to occur in a week or month's time. Recovery takes time. Although these statements are repetitive, they are worth restating.

Robert Callahan, MD[10], a psychiatrist, said it sometimes takes one month of treatment by medications to offset a month of depression. This can be discouraging. However, the alternative is to remain caught up in the funk of depression for a lifetime.

BE PROACTIVE

So what can the individual with a depressive disorder do in the way of self-help? This list of steps one can take to provide some self-help actions identifies examples of activities that the depressed person may explore. These daily and weekly actions assist in overall health and wellness improvement. Before starting any of these steps, consultation with the health care clinician is essential.

STEPS TO TAKE

This list of steps one can take to provide self-help action identifies examples of activities that the depressed person may explore. These daily and weekly actions assist in overall health and wellness improvement. Before starting any of these steps, consultation with the health care clinician is vital.

Get Professional Help

The first step for the individual seeking help for depression is to get professional help from a qualified

---

10   Callahan, Robert M.D., Clinical Director, Joseph W. Johnson Community Mental Health Center, Chattanooga TN (1981)

licensed mental health professional. This essential procedure has been mentioned throughout this book. The person suffering with a depressive disorder and seeking relief from the disorder cannot go it alone.

When talking with a mental health professional the depressed person should describe as accurately as possible the thoughts and behaviors experienced daily. Even if that one does not think a behavior or way of thinking connects with depression, report it to the clinician. Resist telling the clinician what you have self-diagnosed as the problem.

If a physician or psychiatrist has prescribed medications, take them exactly as instructed. Do not take less or more of the prescribed dosage. Allow 2 or 3 weeks to experience the full benefit of the medication and report any suspected adverse reactions to the medication.

When a physician prescribes a medication for the first time for the individual, the physician calls this prescription a "trial dosage." This means the medication is tried to determine its effectiveness in treating the disorder. If it is ineffective, the physician discontinues this trial dosage or substitutes with another medication or increases the strength of dosage as necessary.

Seek out Therapy

Whether it is through individual counseling or in a group setting, psychotherapy may help one deal with depression, both the visible symptoms and the underlying causes of it. Through regular sessions, one learns about the root cause of the depression.

One can then identify healthy changes that can help to cope with and beat depression. These changes may include exploring past relationships, making changes to unhealthy behavior, confronting negative beliefs, and learning to accept things over which one has no control. The skills learned through this process can also help better to handle future crises to avoid another battle with depression.

Learn more by reading related articles.

Knowledge is power. The more a person knows about depression, the more one can accomplish in cooperating with the clinical professional and through self-help activities. Learn all one can about depression. Read books. Check articles on the Internet. Talk with mental health professionals.

One of the worst feelings associated with depression is a sense of helplessness. Depression can leave one feeling as if one has no control over anything in one's life. However, learning as much as one can about one's condition is empowering.

- Anticipate potential problems: Read up on one's medications so you are aware of potential side effects.

- Learn about and practice coping skills. The more skills one has that can help improve one's mood, the better.

- Seek out reputable, trusted doctors and therapists who have written self-help books or run websites or web logs (blogs).

- Get support. Connect with other individuals going through the same thing. Together one might be able to find new ways to cope with depression.

Reach out and stay connected

When one depressed, the tendency is to withdraw and isolate. Even reaching out to close family members and friends can be very difficult. Compound that with the feeling of shame and of neglecting relationships.

Yet social support absolutely is essential to depression recovery. Staying connected to other people and the outside world will make a world of difference in mood and outlook. If it seems that there is no one to which to turn, it is never too late to build new friendships and improve the support network.

- Talk to one person about your feelings
- Help someone else by volunteering
- Have lunch or coffee with a friend
- Ask a loved one to check in with you regularly
- Accompany someone to the movies, a concert, or a small get-together
- Call or email an old friend
- Go for a walk with a workout buddy
- Schedule a weekly dinner date
- Meet new people by taking a class or joining a club
- Confide in a clergy member, teacher, or sports coach

A battle may occur within the depressed person at this primary step in self-help. This step of reaching out runs counter to the symptomatic character of depressive disorders. Finding one person to be the first supportive person will be the challenge.

Look for support from people who make one feel safe and cared for. The person does not have to be able to fix the depression; he or she just needs to be a good listener—someone who will listen attentively and compassionately without being distracted or judgmental.

Make face-time a priority. Phone calls, social media, and texting are great ways to stay in touch, but they do not replace good old-fashioned in-person quality time. The simple act of talking to someone face to face about how one feels can play a big role in lifting the fog of depression and keeping it away.

Find ways to support others. It is nice to receive support, but research shows one gets an even bigger mood boost from providing support one's self. So find ways—both big and small—to help others: Volunteer, be a listening ear for a friend, do something nice for somebody.

Do things that make one feel good—even when one doesn't feel like it

In order to overcome depression, one has to do things that relax and energize. This activity includes following a healthy lifestyle, learning how to manage stress better, setting limits on what one is able to do, and scheduling fun activities into one's day.

While one cannot force oneself to have fun or experience pleasure, one can push oneself to do things, even when one does not feel like it. One might be surprised at how much better one feels once one is not out in the world. Even if one's depression does not lift immediately, the individual gradually feels more upbeat and energetic as one makes time for fun activities.

- Pick up a former hobby or a sport one used to like.
- Express one's self creatively through music, art, or writing.
- Go out with friends.
- Take a day trip to a museum, the mountains, or the ballpark.

Move vigorously during the day—don't sit for more than an hour

When one is depressed, just getting out of bed can seem like a daunting task, let alone working out! However, exercise is a powerful depression fighter—and one of the most important tools in one's recovery arsenal. Research shows that regular exercise can be as effective as medication for relieving depression symptoms. It also helps prevent relapse once one is well.

To get the most benefit, aim for at least 30 minutes of exercise per day. This does not have to be all at once—and it is okay to start small. A 10-minute walk can improve one's mood for two hours. Fatigue will improve if one stick with it.

Starting to exercise can be difficult when one is depressed and exhausted. However, research shows that one's energy levels will improve if one keeps with it. One will be less fatigued, not more, once it is part of one's routine.

Find exercises that are continuous and rhythmic. The most benefits for depression come from rhythmic exercise—such as walking, weight training, swimming, martial arts, or dancing—where one move both one's arms and legs.

Add a mindfulness element, especially if one's depression is rooted in unresolved trauma or fed by obsessive, negative thoughts. Focus on how one's body feels as one move—such as the sensation of one's feet hitting the ground, or the feeling of the wind on one's skin, or the rhythm of one's breathing.

Support one's health with sunshine

Expose one's self to a little sunlight every day. Lack of sunlight can make depression worse. Take a short walk outdoors, have one's coffee outside, enjoy an *al fresco* meal, people-watch on a park bench, or sit out in the garden. Aim for at least 15 minutes of sunlight a day to boost one's mood. If one live somewhere with little winter sunshine, try using a light therapy box.

Sunlight can help boost serotonin levels and improve one's mood. Whenever possible, get outside during daylight hours and expose one's self to the sun. Aim for at least 15 minutes of sunlight a day. Remove sunglasses (but never stare directly at the sun) and use sunscreen as needed.

- Take a walk on one's lunch break, have one's coffee outside, enjoy an al fresco meal, or spend time gardening.

- Double up on the benefits of sunlight by exercising outside. Hike, walk in a local park, or play golf or tennis with a friend.

- Increase the amount of natural light in one's home and workplace by opening blinds and drapes and sitting near windows.

- If one lives somewhere with little winter sunshine, use a light therapy box or lamp.

For some people, the reduced daylight hours of winter lead to a form of depression known as seasonal affective disorder (SAD). SAD can make one feel like a completely different person to who one is in the summer: hopeless, sad, tense, or stressed, with no interest in friends or activities one normally loves. No matter how hopeless one feel, though, there are plenty of things one can do to keep one's mood stable throughout the year.

Relaxation Techniques

Practice relaxation techniques. A daily relaxation practice can help relieve symptoms of depression, reduce stress, and boost feelings of joy and well-being. Try yoga, deep breathing, progressive muscle relaxation, or meditation. Use relaxation tapes or biofeedback.

Get adequate sleep

Sleep Well. Aim for eight hours of sleep. Depression typically involves sleep problems; whether you are sleeping too little or too much, one's mood suffers. Get on a better sleep schedule by learning healthy sleep habits. A good night's sleep can cure many ills, and it just might help one cope with one's depression.

Sleep boosts both one's physical and mental health. Getting enough of it can dramatically increase brain function and improve recovery. However, insomnia and other sleep disorders such as sleep apnea are rather common during depression. Sleep apnea may contribute or cause depression. Talk with one's doctor if one has difficulty sleeping, loud snoring, or waking up gasping for breath.

Eat Healthy

What one eats has a direct impact on how one feels. Reduce one's intake of foods that can adversely affect one's brain and mood, such as caffeine, alcohol, trans fats, and foods with high levels of chemical preservatives or hormones (such as certain meats).

Do not skip meals. Going too long between meals can make one feel irritable and tired, so aim to eat something at least every three to four hours.

Minimize sugar and refined carbohydrates. One may crave sugary snacks, baked goods, or comfort foods such as pasta or French fries, but these "feel-good" foods quickly lead to a crash in mood and energy. Aim to cut out as much of these foods as possible.

Boost one's B and D_3 vitamins.

Deficiencies in B vitamins such as folic acid and B_{12} can trigger depression. To get more, take a B-complex vitamin supplement or eat more citrus fruit, leafy greens, beans, chicken, and eggs.

Challenge negative thinking

Does one feel powerless or weak? That bad things happen and there's not much one can do about it? That one's situation is hopeless. Depression puts a negative spin on everything, including the way one see one's self and one's expectations for the future.

When these types of thoughts overwhelm you, it is important to remind oneself that this is the depression talking. These irrational, pessimistic attitudes—known as *cognitive distortions*—are not realistic.

When one really examines them, they don't hold up. Even so, they can be tough to give up. Just telling one's self to "think positive" will not cut it. Often, they are part of a lifelong pattern of thinking that has become so automatic one is not even completely aware of it. Negative, unrealistic ways of thinking that fuel depression may include:

- All-or-nothing thinking – Looking at things in black-or-white categories, with no middle ground ("If I fall short of perfection, I'm a total failure.")

- Overgeneralization – Generalizing from a single negative experience, expecting it to hold true forever ("I can't do anything right.")

- The mental filter – Ignoring positive events and focusing on the negative. Noticing the one thing that went wrong, rather than all the things that went right.

- Diminishing the positive – Coming up with reasons why positive events do not count ("She said she had a good time on our date, but I think she was just being nice.")

- Emotional reasoning – Believing that the way one feel reflects reality ("I feel like such a loser. I really am no good!")

- Jumping to conclusions – Making negative interpretations without actual evidence. One act like a mind reader ("He must think I'm pathetic") or a fortuneteller ("I'll be stuck in this dead end job forever.")

- Perfectionism: 'Should' and 'should-not' – Holding one's self to a strict list of what one should and shouldn't do, and beating one's self up if one don't live up to one's rules.

- Labeling – Labeling oneself based on mistakes and perceived shortcomings ("I'm a failure; an idiot; a loser." "I'm scum.")

- Once one identify the destructive thoughts patterns that one default to, one can start to challenge them with questions such as:

- "What's the evidence that this thought is true? Not true?"

- "What would I tell a friend who had this thought?"

- "Is there another way of looking at the situation or an alternate explanation?"

- "How might I look at this situation if I didn't have depression?"

- As one cross-examines one's negative thoughts, one may be surprised at how quickly they crumble. In the process, one will develop a more balanced perspective.

Develop a "wellness tool kit" to deal with depression

Come up with a list of things that one can accomplish for a quick mood boost. The more "tools" one has for coping with depression, the better. Try to implement a few of these ideas each day, even if one is feeling good.

- Spend some time in nature
- List what one like about yourself
- Read a good book
- Watch a funny movie or TV show
- Take a long, hot bath
- Take care of a few small tasks
- Play with a pet
- Talk to friends or family face-to-face
- Listen to music
- Do something spontaneous

Keep a journal

A journal, calendar, or daily log of some sort can help one see how some days are better than others are. Jot down what one did, whom one saw, and anything else that one thinks would be helpful to look at again later. Smartphone apps can also be helpful in tracking one's symptoms and triggers.

The depressed person might choose to make the journal comprehensive. Especially helpful with individuals with other medical conditions such as diabetes or obesity among others, the journal might be helpful to the clinical professional in determining how conditions might interrelate. Many people, who journal about their depression, also record their weight, blood sugar results, and exercises performed during the day. Some even journal what they ate and when.

Avoid Drugs and Alcohol

Unfortunately, the all-too-common misconception is that drugs and alcohol will make depression better. While such substances may help the depressed one forget the depressive condition temporarily, drugs and alcohol can actually make depression worse. On top of this, many antidepressant drugs react negatively with drugs and alcohol. These substances can put one in danger. If one has a problem resisting either drugs or alcohol, the therapist or physician should be informed and appropriate actions taken.

Look at alternative medicines.

Some herbal remedies and supplements that may help treat one's depression. These alternatives or supplements require discussion with a physician before undertaken.

These include:

- Folate, a B vitamin, may help antidepressant medications work more efficiently. When one's body does not have enough folate, it may have a slower-than-normal response to antidepressant medicines.

- Omega-3 fatty acids are heart-healthy fats that may ease symptoms of depression. Cold-water fish are chock-full of omega-3s, as are flaxseed, flax oil, walnuts, and algae supplements.

- St. John's wort, also known as *Hypericum perforatum*, is an herb used for centuries to treat many conditions, including depression. While it may help, it is not an FDA-approved treatment for depression.

- At times, B_{12} might also be supportive of overall well being and in the treatment of depressive disorders.

WHAT FAMILY MEMBERS CAN DO

This all sounds good. Much of the self-help list suggested above requires the depressed individual to "do something." Yet the very nature of depression (the Catch-22) is that the depressed person does not have the ability to "do something. Reaching out to others for support and assistance can be a daunting task.

Often the most effective and helpful way a friend or family member can support a person with depression is to reach out to the depressed individual instead, rather than expecting the depressed one to reach out. "If you need me, just call," or "Why didn't you call me if you were in such a difficult time," are unhelpful statements and at worst are justifications for not reaching out to the other person. These statements may at best clearly show a true misunderstanding of the nature of depression.

Too often, we know depression is a serious medical situation but we regard it in much the same was as a broken leg or influenza. We think the person has the mental ability to know when and how to reach out to someone when that one needs assistance. This is not the case with a person suffering with a depressive disorder.

Some of the common and characteristic symptoms of depression have to do with mental function—inability to concentrate, inability to make decisions (good or bad), inability to remember things. Furthermore, social isolation and withdrawal from social contact with others has a common manifestation in depressed individuals. Add to that the sense of helplessness and hopelessness and not wanting to bother.

These factors usually preclude the depressed individual from reaching out for help in time of need. It is extremely useful for the friend or family member to take the initiative. If that friend or family member does not reach out to the depressed one, the contact will most probably not occur.

Because of the nature of the illness, the depressed one has not the motivation or the energy to do the reaching out. It is important that friends and family stay in contact with and involved in the life of the one suffering from depression.

With that said, here is a partial list of ways a family member of friend may assist and support one with a depressive disorder.

HOW TO HELP

Learn to recognize the symptoms of depression

Study the symptoms for depression found in the table in Chapter 2. Become familiar with these symptomatic behaviors and look for them in the one you suspect is depressed.

Learn more by reading related articles.

Visit the library or search on line for authentic articles from reliable sources on depression. Learn as much about depression and how to support or intervene as possible.

Help the depressed person seek out therapy

Be available to the person struggling with depression by providing that one transportation to a therapy session. Be available, but don't coerce.

Help the depressed individual to move vigorously during the day

- Become a workout partner for the depressed individual.
- Take the depressed person on your daily walks. Pick that one up.
- Drive the person to the gym or fitness center.

Help the depressed person do things that make one feel good—even when that one doesn't feel like it.

- Encourage taking up a former hobby or a sport one used to like.
- Promote self creatively through music, art, or writing.
- Take the person out with friends.
- Take the depressed person on a day trip to a museum, the mountains, or the ballpark.

Reach out to the depressed person daily and stay connected to them.

A battle may occur within the depressed person at this primary step in self-help; again, it is the Catch-22.

- Be available to talk to the depressed one about emotions and feelings. Mostly, just listen without attempting to explain.

- Take the depressed one with you to someone else by volunteering.

- Have lunch or coffee with the person.

- Check in with the depressed person regularly.

- Accompany the person who is depressed to the movies, a concert, or a small get-together. Pick the person up. Do not ask him or her to meet you.

- Be a workout friend and go for a walk with the one who is depressed.

- Schedule a weekly dinner date with the depressed person. Again, pick that person up. Relying on the person to meet you probably is not an effective strategy.

- Take the depressed one to meet new people by taking a class or joining a club.

Help the person with depression by encouraging a healthy lifestyle.

Sunshine is essential, especially with those individuals afflicted with Seasonal Affective Disorder (SAD). Dropping by regularly to take the depressed person out into the sunshine can be a very effective weapon against the isolation and the deprivation of sunlight. A trip to a shopping mall or a walk in the park is a good starting point. Perhaps a picnic in the outdoors in good weather can be useful, as well.

Healthy eating is essential in the recovery from depression. Again, because of brain function problems, a person with depression may not eat healthy meals. Lack of energy, lack of motivation, inability to develop healthy menu plans, and problems shopping are common among many depressed people. The friend or family member can be of great assistance here.

Help the depressed one to develop a week's menus for all meals, including healthy snacks. Then take the person shopping for weekly groceries. Remember many food stores give senior discounts to the elderly on Wednesdays.

Help by also preparing some meals, either for immediate consumption or refrigerated for eating later during the week. Remember that the meal planning and the shopping for (and putting away) groceries is only part of the work. Lack of energy and lack of motivation can prevent these efforts from being effective. Food in the refrigerator may spoil if the depressed person does not have or cannot find the energy to prepare meals.

Help with household chores.

This could well be the most important of all the helpful actions to take. Looking at a dirty house reinforces the depression. Lack of energy and lack of motivation once again play a big part of the broken lifestyle. Not only does completing chores around the house—cleaning, laundry, repairs, and maintenance, even carrying out the garbage, not only help with a healthy environment, it gives a fresh view to a person with depression. Not all seems so helpless after all.

Do not be shy about going into a dirty house. The depressed person may say it isn't needed or even wanted, but deep inside there usually is a sense of relief and hope. Just remember, what occurs and the condition of the house must remain a matter of privacy.

Not all friends need to know. The person already feels badly about the condition and does not need additional feelings of shame. In four words, "Keep Your Mouth Shut!"

SUMMARY

Talking with one's doctor or therapist and getting medical attention is the first step to beating depression. Eight tips may help one to feel better too. Always consult the physician before starting any of suggested regimens. Counselors must refer their patients who are considering self-help activity to their physician for consultation.

For those who are family members or friends of the person struggling with depression, the important thing to remember is the need to take the initiative. Waiting for the depressed person to seek out help will result in no reaching out. That is the nature of most depressive conditions. Go there. Be there. Listen.

REVIEW QUESTIONS

(written or discussion)

1. The first step in resolving depression is to

   _____.

2. Always consult the physician when _____

   _____.

3. Counselors must refer their clients who are considering _____ to their physician.

4. For family and friends of the depressed person, it is important to _____ on that person's behalf.

5. Waiting for the depressed person to seek out help will result in _____.

CLASS DISCUSSION

What is the best way for an individual to battle depression? What should family and friends do to help and support the depressed person?

Case Study of "Mr. Bailey"

Mr. Bailey lived in a small town located in a rural county in a state in the southeastern United States of America. He was widowed and lived alone in his home. He had one brother living, who was 3 years younger, and a sister 2 years older than he. Mr. Bailey was in his early 60s in age. He was tall, lean, and graying.

After heart surgery, because he lived alone and had no one to care for him during recovery, Mr. Bailey was placed in the local nursing home. At first, he made good progress physically. However, Mr. Bailey became socially withdrawn, helpless in his personal care, and slovenly in appearance, often defecating or urinating in his pants. His speech began to slur and finally he only made animated vocal sounds.

A consulting geriatric social worker in private practice had a contract with the nursing home and was asked to see Mr. Bailey. The social worker was taken to Mr. Bailey's room by the nursing staff who curiously waited just outside the door to listen in on the interview.

The social worker approached Mr. Bailey, who was sitting in a chair, head down, staring at the floor. Mr. Bailey smelled of urine. The social worker knelt in front of Mr. Bailey and introduced himself. The conversation with something like this:

Social Worker (SW): Hi, Mr. Bailey (MB). I am (name withheld). I am a social worker and was asked to talk with you today. So, tell me how are you today?

MB: (saying nothing, continued to stare at the floor.)

SW: I see. You don't feel like talking to me right now. That's all right. But the nursing home staff had some concerns about you. They say you are recovering from your surgery very well but that you don't seem to be very responsive to them or the other patients here. Could you tell me what that is about?

MB: (no response, still staring at the floor)

SW: I understand your brother and your sister came to visit you yesterday. What did you think about their visit?

MB: (made a sound that sounded like pfftt.)

SW: Oh, I see. So, the visit didn't go well for you. Is there a problem between you and your brother and sister? Are you upset with them for some reason?

MB: (not speaking, looked up and directly into the eyes of the social worker)

SW: Ah, so why don't you tell me about that.

MB: (Mumbling) (pointed at his upper left chest).

SW: OK, Mr. Bailey, I only understood one word, heart, but that's ok. You are talking about your heart. Are you concerned about your heart?

MB: rhummbachifoonurrsee heart semulcopohlallelaway die.

SW: You are talking about your heart and dying? You think you are going to die? But the nurses have told me you are recovering from your heart surgery and your heart is going to be fine.

MB: Parcommacomdusilahcantu heart. Repotagrabble here wayto die.

SW: Oh, are you telling me that because of your heart you are waiting to die? Well, Mr. Bailey, we all die, don't we? But the doctor said you are not going to die right now because of your heart problem. He said you will be fine.

MB: (straightened up in his chair, still looking intensely at the social worker, with clearly visible tension in his muscles)

SW: Mr. Bailey, do you think you have been placed here in the nursing home because you are dying? That is not true at all. Your brother and sister said they were concerned that no one was able to stay with you during your recovery from the surgery, and that because of that, you had to be in a nursing home until you were strong enough to take care of yourself, prepare meals, walk about without assistance, and do the chores around your house.

MB: Oh

SW: Yeah, so you see, MB, no one thinks you are dying except you. You have just misunderstood. I am sorry no one better explained to you what is going on and why you were here.

MB: Thank you.

SW: You are very welcome, sir. Tell me what you are thinking now.

MB: I thought nursing homes is where you go to die.

SW: No, Mr. Bailey. Of course, some people in nursing homes do die there, but this place is where nurses assist you to get well. That's why it is called a nursing home. It is your temporary home while you get proper nursing care while you get well.

MB: Oh. Then I am not here to die?

SW: No, Mr. Bailey. You are here until you can take care of yourself without assistance. We could start right now, if you would like. Why don't you stand up and go take a shower and put on some clean clothes? (SW stretching out arms to assist his standing)

MB: (taking SW hands, pulls himself to the standing position) I never thought I would ever do this again.

SW: You're fine Mr. Bailey. Now let's walk over and see what clothes you would like to wear after your shower.

At this point, a nurse's aid came quickly into to the room and started to look for clean clothes for Mr. Bailey to put on.

SW: No, let's allow Mr. Bailey to make his own selection. He needs to start making decisions and doing things for himself.

The nurse's aid quickly stepped back as Mr. Bailey selected his attire for the day, set them aside on the bed, and removing his soiled clothes, took a shower by himself, with the nurse's aid and social worker standing by outside in the event Mr. Bailey fell. But he didn't.

A week later the social worker returned to the nursing home to see another resident and found Mr. Bailey and several other men sitting in rocking chairs on the porch, joking and talking and carrying on happily.

The point of this true-life example (with the name changed, of course) shows that life circumstances, emotional and physical stress, and misunderstanding all contribute to the development of a depressive episode. Mr. Bailey had a physical trauma in the heart surgery. He had been in the nursing home about 5 weeks, and his body was clearly responding well to the care he was receiving.

However, Mr. Bailey did not understand or was not told why he was in the nursing home. Perhaps the family and staff assumed he knew what nursing homes were for. Yet, Mr. Bailey was of a generation of the past where hospitals and nursing homes were places one went to die.

As a result of this occurrence, Mr. Bailey had become fearful of dying and angry at his brother and sister for shutting him away to die at the nursing home and not at his own home. He became withdrawn, and developed feelings of hopelessness, helplessness, and despair. Mr. Bailey gave up. He lost his resolve. He mentally and emotionally deteriorated.

One consideration must be mentioned. In this book, a point is made that people with depression need a friend or family member to reach out and help at times. It is crucial that such help occurs in a manner that a message is sent, in some way, that tells the depressed one that she is not incapable but that the helper wants to support rather than take care of the depressed one.

Summary

Depression is real, complicated, and greatly misunderstood. Depression is painful. A significant amount of disharmony, hurt, and anger may result. Criticism and unmet expectations create difficulty in relationships. Depression can make everyone involved in it unhappy and miserable. Depression affects family life, community efforts at resolving a number of local issues, and policy decisions in the arenas of public health, mental health, economics, social welfare, and politics.

Causal factors for depression may be four-fold. One, two, three or all four factors may be at play in the condition. These four causal factors are physical trauma, biological change, and emotional upset and genetic make up. Physical trauma—a broken bone, or a hormonal shift may cause a state of depression in an individual. Depressive disorders require a comprehensive clinical, social, and medical evaluation to determine treatment, care, and support options.

However, recent research has found certain genetic defects seem to be causal to depression and other more severe disorders such as schizophrenia. This break-through in science allows a greater understanding of why some people do not fully respond to various treatment interventions and do not totally recover from a major depressive episode. We seem to have far to go.

Depression may actually paralyze a person's cognitive and emotional functioning. It can drain one physically of energy and mobility. Depression is one of the most common mental disorders in the United States.

The World Health Organization has characterized depression as one of the most disabling disorders in the world. Depression can happen at any age, but often begins in late adolescence or early adulthood. Many chronic mood and anxiety disorders in adults begin as high levels of anxiety in children.

Depression in midlife or older adults can occur with other serious medical illnesses, such as diabetes, cancer, heart disease, and Parkinson's disease. Sometimes medications taken for these physical illnesses may cause side effects that contribute to depression. Depression may also appear like symptoms of dementia and Alzheimer's disease.

THREE DOMAINS OF DEVELOPMENT AND FUNCTION

People develop and function in what we call three domains—the Affective Domain, the Behavioral Domain, and the Cognitive Domain. These domains represent the way individuals feel, behave, and think. The Affective Domain is the domain of moods, attitudes, and emotions. The Behavioral Domain centers in the behaviors one presents. The Cognitive Domain is the domain of the mind.

These are the ABC's of the self. Affective is feeling, Behavioral is doing, and Cognitive is thinking. The effects of these three domains on the self extend into all areas of human development and function. The battle with depression is largely the battle for cognition.

MAKING A DIAGNOSIS

The Diagnostic and Statistical Manual of Mental Disorders (DSM) is the handbook used by health care professionals in the United States and much of the world as the authoritative guide to the diagnosis of mental disorders. DSM contains descriptions, symptoms, and other criteria for diagnosing mental disorders. The American Psychiatric Association publishes it. Currently the DSM is in its fifth edition and known commonly as the DSM-5.

The symptoms of depression are many. Not everyone has all these symptoms. We do not always recognize certain symptoms or behaviors as symptoms of a depressive disorder.

Depression is a syndrome—a disorder having a set of symptoms. Having one or two of these symptoms from time to time does not indicate depression. Persistent occurrence or reoccurrence of several of these symptoms may be indicative of clinical depression.

HOW DEPRESSION WORKS

The brain has billions of nerve cells. They do not actually touch. Neurotransmitters carry messages back and forth.

When a person has depression, the brain energy level may deplete. Just as with an automobile's electrical system, our bodies also have "electrical systems." Just as in an automobile, each component part of the body's electrical system has a vital part to play in the proper functioning of our bodies.

The brain, our energy source, controls memory, mood, and movement. Energy from the brain moves from nerve to nerve in the form of neurotransmitters located in the synapses. When the brain or the synapse is deficient in neurotransmitters, depression occurs.

A neurotransmitter is a chemical substance that released at the end of a nerve fiber by the arrival of a nerve impulse. It diffuses across the synapse or junction, causing the transfer of the impulse to another nerve fiber, a muscle fiber, or some other structure. Nerve fibers release neurotransmitters from synaptic vesicles in synapses into the synaptic cleft and received by receptors on the target cells.

Causes of depression categorize as biological differences, brain chemistry emotional upset, physical trauma, and genetic mutation, inherited traits, and life events. Three key common emotions – anger, fear, and guilt, may trigger depression. In disorders such as depression, diabetes, and high blood pressure, a combination of genetic changes seem to predispose some people to become ill. More than one genetic factor may be responsible for the predisposition of certain individuals for the condition.

TYPES OF DEPRESSIVE DISORDERS

Two diagnostic types of depression—persistent depressive disorder and major depressive disorder or clinical depression, exist. Depression at times occurs in other diagnosed diseases or disorders. Depression may go undiagnosed or misdiagnosed due to lack of clear and sufficient information about a patient's behavior.

Depression does not go away for everyone. Major depression can occur from one generation to the next in different families. It can also affect people with no family history of the illness.

A small percentage of people remain who can talk about their issues, express their feelings, take very good care of themselves emotionally, even take medication and have a great life, and still be depressed throughout their lives. To people around them, these individuals seem healthy and alive even while struggling deep inside. The hope remains that even this type of depression remains treatable. A meaningful life may occur.

Because the mind is part of the illness, people usually do not see the dynamics of this debilitating and paralyzing condition. Exasperation, resentment or animosity can override any notions of patience and empathy. Successive major depressive episodes make it more certain that additional episodes will occur.

In comparison to other debilitating, painful, potentially fatal illnesses or injuries, severe depression is unique in how it affects one's mind, behavior, personality, and thought processes. Some other forms of depression include perinatal depression, seasonal affective disorder, psychotic depression, and cyclothymic disorder. Examples of other types of depressive disorders newly added to the diagnostic classification of DSM-5 include disruptive mood dysregulation disorder (diagnosed in children and adolescents) and premenstrual dysphoric disorder (PMDD).

CASE STUDIES

Twelve actual case situations demonstrate the real stuff, the actual description of depressive disorder from the perspective of the one who is depressed. These case studies reflect internalized anger, fear, and guilt— not always obviously displayed. The studies show the hopelessness, the isolation, and the despair of individuals who suffer from a depressive disorder.

The studies provide a critical view of how depression distorts or confuses cognitive processes. A majority of those interacting with a depressed person cannot understand such cognition difficulties. The cry for help often goes unanswered.

The interview with James demonstrates the thinking, behavior, mood, and attitude of one with a depressive disorder. Candid responses provide the opportunity to get inside the head of one person— and only that one person. The interview reveals some distorted thinking by James about his depression and his life circumstances. Interviews such as the one with James reveal additional insights about depressive disorders.

SUPPORT AND SERVICES

Depression is treatable. Support is available from a number of local, state, and national organizations that provide information, financial assistance, and assistance for coping and advocacy. It is important to know that the depressed individual and the family are not alone.

However, many individuals suffering with depression have impaired cognitive processes. Because of this fact, these individuals may not be able personally to access these resources or to seek services from them. A referral to another agency or service is insufficient in many cases.

Therefore, the role of the competent social worker is more than intake and referral or psychotherapy. It is for the clinical social worker more than just counsel and referral. Social workers must be willing and available to their clients and patients to contact these resources and arrange services for the individuals in their caseload or practice.

Social workers must always retain their function as grass roots change agents. Too often social work roles in private practice and in mental health treatment facilities have lost that grass roots aspect of change agent. Social workers must be willing to make that telephone call to another agency, to advocate for their clients, and to be more than a therapist or a referral source. Sometimes action is required.

For the depressed individual, talking with one's doctor or therapist and getting medical attention is the first step to beating depression. Eight tips may help one to feel better too. Always consult the physician before starting any of suggested regimens. Counselors must refer their patients who are considering self-help activity to their physician for consultation.

For those who are family members or friends of the person struggling with depression, the important thing to remember is the need to take the initiative. Waiting for the depressed person to seek out help will result in no reaching out. That is the nature of most depressive conditions. *Go there. Be there. Listen.*

CLASS DISCUSSION

1. What is depression?
2. What are the most common forms of the disorder?
3. How does depression manifest itself in an individual? What causes depression?
4. How does depression work?
5. What effect does depression have on the attitude, behavior, mood, and thinking of the person with the disorder?
6. How does a depressive disorder affect family, friends, coworkers, and others interacting with the depressed person?
7. How does one seek help for depression in oneself or in another person?
8. How is depression treated?
9. What are some new trends in the treatment of depression?

A Word Of Appreciation

The author expresses his heartfelt appreciation to the individual members of the K-POP boy band BTS of Seoul, Korea for their support and contributions to this work. Their comments, both in direct communication with the author and in a media interview, were invaluable in understanding that depression is a universal issue that is neither gender nor age specific. The reader will find their comments and quotations throughout the book. Thanks, men.

Jeon Jungkook (Jungkook)

Jung Hoseok (J-Hope)

Kim Taehyung (V)

Kim Seok-Jin (Jin)

Kim Namjoon (RM)

Min Yoongi (Suga)

Park Jimin (Jimin)

Appendix 1

WORD LIST

Students and learners should be able to define these terms upon examination. These words occur frequently not only in social work settings but also in psychiatric nursing, psychology, psychiatry, nutrition, physical therapy, pharmacology, and biochemistry. Make them a part of your professional vocabulary.

A social worker must speak the language of the other person. That other person may mean a client, someone in poverty, a depressed person, a person in business, construction, manufacturing, or retail. That other person may be a mental health professional or a nursing specialist.

The social worker, as a change and communications agent, must have the vocabulary to speak the language of many occupations, professions, vocations, cultures, and clients. Unless the social worker can speak the language of the other person, communication may not occur, or miscommunication creates difficulties in providing services and treatment to the individual client.

A

Abnormal psychology The area of psychological investigation concerned with understanding the nature of individual pathologies of mind, mood, and behavior.

Acetylcholine. A compound that occurs throughout the nervous system, in which it functions as a neurotransmitter.

Acquisition The stage in a classical conditioning experiment during which the conditioned response is first elicited by the conditioned stimulus.

Acquisition The stage in a classical conditioning experiment during which the conditioned response is first elicited by the conditioned stimulus.

Acute stress A transient state of arousal with typically clear onset and offset patterns.

Addiction A condition in which the body requires a drug in order to function without physical and psychological reactions to its absence; often the outcome of tolerance and dependence.

Adrenaline. A hormone secreted by the adrenal glands, especially in conditions of stress, increasing rates of blood circulation, breathing, and carbohydrate metabolism and preparing muscles for exertion

Affect. A concept used in psychology to describe the experience of feeling or emotion. The term **affect** (philosophy) takes on a different meaning in other fields. The word also refers sometimes to **affect** display, which is "a facial, vocal, or gestural behavior that serves as an indicator of **affect**" (APA 2006).

Alkyl. Of or denoting a hydrocarbon radical derived from an alkane by removal of a hydrogen atom.

Alzheimer's disease. Progressive mental deterioration that can occur in middle or old age, due to generalized degeneration of the brain. It is the most common cause of premature senility.

Amino acid. A simple organic compound containing both a carboxyl ($-COOH$) and an amino ($-NH_2$) group

Amygdala The part of the limbic system that controls emotion, aggression, and the formation of emotional memory.

Androgen. A male sex hormone, such as testosterone

Anterior. Nearer the front, especially situated in the front of the body or nearer to the head.

Anterior pituitary gland. A major organ of the endocrine system (also called the adenohypophysis or pars anterior), is the glandular, anterior lobe that together with the posterior lobe (posterior pituitary, or the neurohypophysis) makes up the pituitary gland (hypophysis).

Anticipatory coping Efforts made in advance of a potentially stressful event to overcome, reduce, or tolerate the imbalance between perceived demands and available resources

Anxiety. A nervous disorder characterized by a state of excessive uneasiness and apprehension, typically with compulsive behavior or panic attacks, caused by the preconscious recognition that a repressed conflict is about to emerge into consciousness.

Anxiety disorders Mental disorders marked by physiological arousal, feelings of tension, and intense apprehension without apparent reason.

Association cortex The parts of the cerebral cortex in which many high-level brain processes occur.

Attachment Emotional relationship between a child and the "regular caregiver

Attention A state of focused awareness on a subset of the available perceptual information

Attitude The learned, relatively stable tendency to respond to people, concepts, and events in an evaluative way

Axial. Of, forming, or relating to an axis. Around an axis.

Axon. The long threadlike part of a nerve cell along which impulses are conducted from the cell body to other cells

B

Behavior modification The systematic use of principles of learning to increase the frequency of desired behaviors and/or decrease the frequency of problem behaviors

Behavioral therapy. An umbrella term for types of *therapy* that treat mental health disorders. This form of *therapy* seeks to identify and help change potentially self-destructive or unhealthy *behaviors*. The focus of treatment is often on current problems and how to change them

Behaviorist perspective The psychological perspective primarily concerned with observable behavior that can be objectively recorded and with the relationships of observable behavior to environmental stimuli.

Biofeedback A self-regulatory technique by which an individual acquires voluntary control over nonconscious biological processes.

Biomedical therapies Treatments for psychological disorders that alter brain functioning with chemical or physical interventions such as drug therapy, surgery, or electroconvulsive therapy.

Biopsychosocial model A model of health and illness that suggests that links among the nervous system, the immune system, behavioral styles, cognitive processing, and environmental factors can put people at risk for illness.

Bi-Polar See Cyclothymia

C

Cannon-Bard theory of emotion A theory stating that an "emotional stimulus produces two co-occurring reactions — arousal and experience of emotion — that do not cause each other."

CAT Scan. An X-ray image made using computerized axial tomography. See also Electroencephalogram (EEG) and Magnetic resonance imaging (*MRI*).

Central nervous system (CNS) The part of the nervous system consisting of the brain and spinal cord

Cerebellum The region of the brain attached to the brain stem that controls motor coordination, posture, and balance as well as the ability to learn control of body movements

Cerebrum. The principal and most anterior part of the brain in vertebrates, located in the front area of the skull and consisting of two hemispheres, left and right, separated by a fissure. It is responsible for the integration of complex sensory and neural functions and the initiation and coordination of voluntary activity in the body

Cholesterol. A compound of the sterol type found in most body tissues Cholesterol and its derivatives are important constituents of cell membranes and precursors of other steroid compounds, but a high proportion in the blood of low-density lipoprotein (which transports cholesterol to the tissues) is associated with an increased risk of coronary heart disease

Circadian rhythm. Often referred to as the "body clock," the circadian rhythm is a cycle that tells our bodies when to sleep, rise, eat—regulating many physiological processes. Environmental cues, like sunlight and temperature affect this internal body clock

Classical conditioning A type of learning in which a behavior (conditioned response) comes to be elicited by a stimulus (conditioned stimulus) that has acquired its power through an association with a biologically significant stimulus (unconditioned stimulus).

Client-centered therapy A humanistic approach to treatment that emphasizes the healthy psychological growth of the individual; based on the assumption that all people share the basic tendency of human nature toward self-actualization.

Clinical psychologist An individual who has earned a doctorate in psychology and whose training is in the assessment and treatment of psychological problems

Clinical social worker A mental health professional whose specialized training prepares him or her to consider the social context of people's problems

Closure A perceptual organizing process that leads individuals to see incomplete figures as complete.

Cognition. The mental action or process of acquiring knowledge and understanding through thought, experience, and the senses. A result of this; a perception, sensation, notion, or intuition

Cognitive. See Cognition

Cognitive distortion. Are simply ways that our mind convinces us of something that isn't really true. These inaccurate thoughts are usually used to reinforce negative thinking or emotions — telling ourselves things that sound rational and accurate, but really only serve to keep us feeling bad about ourselves

Cognitive therapy. A type of psychotherapy in which negative patterns of thought about the self and the world are challenged in order to alter unwanted behavior patterns or treat mood disorders such as depression

Computerized axial tomography. A form of tomography in which a computer controls the motion of the X-ray source and detectors, processes the data, and produces the image.

Conditioning The ways in which events, stimuli, and behavior become associated with one another

Cortex. The outer layer of the cerebrum (the *cerebral cortex*), composed of folded gray matter and playing an important role in consciousness

Cortical. Relating to the outer layer of the cerebrum

Counseling psychologist Psychologist who specializes in providing guidance in areas such as vocational selection, school problems, drug abuse, and marital conflict.

Cyclothymia. A mental state characterized by marked swings of mood between depression and elation; bipolar disorder

D

Decision making The process of choosing between alternatives; selecting or rejecting available options.

Delusion. An idiosyncratic belief or impression firmly maintained despite contradiction by what is generally accepted as reality or rational argument, typically a symptom of mental disorder. See also Hallucination and Illusion.

Dementia. A chronic or persistent disorder of the mental processes caused by brain disease or injury and marked by memory disorders, personality changes, and impaired reasoning.

Depression. Feelings of severe despondency and dejection. Depression is a common and serious medical illness that negatively affects how one feels, the way one thinks, and how one acts. Fortunately, it is also treatable. *Depression* causes feelings of sadness and/or a loss of interest in activities once enjoyed.

Dialectics. The art of investigating or discussing the truth of opinions. A dialogue, a debate, a discussion

Diffusion. The spreading of something more widely

Dopamine. A compound present in the body as a neurotransmitter and a precursor of other substances including epinephrine

Dopamine Dysphoria. See Dopamine dysregulation syndrome (DDS)

Dopamine dysregulation syndrome (DDS) consists of a series of complications such as compulsive use of dopaminergic medications, aggressive or hypomanic behaviors during excessive use, and withdrawal states characterized by dysphoria and anxiety, caused by long-term dopaminergic treatment in patients with Parkinson's

Dysphoria. A state of unease or generalized dissatisfaction with life

Dysthymia. Persistent mild depression.

E

Electroencephalogram (EEG) A recording of the electrical activity of the brain. See also CAT Scan and Magnetic resonance imaging (*MRI*).

Emotion A complex pattern of changes, including physiological arousal, feelings, cognitive processes, and behavioral reactions, made in response to a situation perceived to be personally significant.

Emotional intelligence Type of intelligence defined as the abilities to perceive, appraise, and express emotions accurately and appropriately, to use emotions to facilitate thinking, to understand and analyze emotions, to use emotional knowledge effectively, and to regulate one's emotions to promote both emotional and intellectual growth.

Endocrine. Relating to or denoting glands that secrete hormones or other products directly into the blood.

Endocrine System. The *endocrine* system is the collection of glands that produce hormones that regulate metabolism, growth and development, tissue function, sexual function, reproduction, sleep, and mood, among other things. The endocrine system is the collection of glands of an organism that secrete hormones directly into the circulatory system to be carried towards distant target organs.
In humans, the major endocrine glands include the pineal gland, testes, thyroid gland, parathyroid gland, and adrenal glands. In vertebrates, the hypothalamus is the neural control center for all endocrine systems.

Ester. An organic compound made by replacing the hydrogen of an acid by an alkyl or other organic group. Many naturally occurring fats and essential oils are esters of fatty acids.

Estradiol. A form of the hormone estrogen. It's also called 17 beta-*estradiol*. The ovaries, breasts, and adrenal glands make *estradiol*. During pregnancy, the placenta also makes *estradiol*.

Estrogen. Any of a group of steroid hormones that promote the development and maintenance of female characteristics of the body. Such hormones are also produced artificially for use in oral contraceptives or to treat menopausal and menstrual disorders.

Etiology The causes of, or factors related to, the development of a disorder.

F

Fight-or-flight response A sequence of internal activities triggered when an organism is faced with a threat; prepares the body for combat and struggle or for running away to safety; recent evidence suggests that the response is characteristic only of males.

Fixation A state in which a person remains attached to objects or activities more appropriate for an earlier stage of psychosexual development.

Fluid intelligence The aspect of intelligence that involves the ability to see complex relationships and solve problems.

Frontal Lobe. Each of the paired lobes of the brain lying immediately behind the forehead, including areas concerned with behavior, learning, personality, and voluntary movement.

Frustration-aggression hypothesis According to this hypothesis, frustration occurs in situations in which people are prevented or blocked from attaining their goals; a rise in frustration then leads to a greater probability of aggression.

G

Gamma-amino butyric acid (GABA) A neurotransmitter that sends chemical messages through the brain and the nervous system, and is involved in regulating communication between brain cells. The role of **GABA** is to inhibit or reduce the activity of the neurons or nerve cells.

Generalized anxiety disorder An anxiety disorder in which an individual feels anxious and worried most of the time for at least six months when not threatened by any specific danger or object.

Gland. An organ in the human or animal body that secretes particular chemical substances for use in the body or for discharge into the surroundings

Glycoprotein. Any of a class of proteins that have carbohydrate groups attached to the polypeptide chain. Also called *glycopeptide*.

Glycoprotein hormone. Are the most complex molecules with *hormonal* activity. They include three pituitary *hormones*, the gonadotropins follicle-stimulating hormone (FSH; follitropin) and luteinizing *hormone* (LH; lutropin) as well as thyroid-stimulating *hormone* (TSH; thyrotropin) (1).

H

Hallucination. An experience involving the apparent perception of something not present. See also Delusion and Illusion.

Heredity The biological transmission of traits from parents to offspring.

Hierarchy of needs Maslow's view that basic human motives form a hierarchy and that the needs at each level of the hierarchy must be satisfied before the next level can be achieved; these needs progress from basic biological needs to the need for transcendence.

Hippocampal. See Hippocampus

Hippocampal neurogenesis. A unique form of neural circuit plasticity that results in the generation of new neurons in the dentate gyrus throughout life

Hippocampus. A small region of the brain that forms part of the limbic system and is primarily associated with memory and spatial navigation.

Homeostasis. The tendency toward a relatively stable equilibrium between interdependent elements, especially as maintained by physiological processes.

Hormone. A regulatory substance produced in an organism and transported in tissue fluids such as blood or sap to stimulate specific cells or tissues into action. Hormones can be categorized into three distinct groups according to their chemical composition. The three types of hormones are steroid hormones, *peptide hormones* and amino acid derivatives. The different types of hormones will have different mechanisms of action due to their distinct chemical properties.

Human behavior genetics The area of study that evaluates the genetic component of individual differences in behaviors and traits.

Human-potential movement The therapy movement that encompasses all those practices and methods that release the potential of the average human being for greater levels of performance and greater richness of experience.

Humanistic perspective A psychological model that emphasizes an individual's phenomenal world and inherent capacity for making rational choices and developing to maximum potential.

Hypothalamus. A region of the forebrain below the thalamus that coordinates both the autonomic nervous system and the activity of the pituitary, controlling body temperature, thirst, hunger, and other homeostatic systems, and involved in sleep and emotional activity.

I

Illusion An experience of a stimulus pattern in a manner that is demonstrably incorrect but shared by others in the same perceptual environment. See also delusion and hallucination.

Implosion therapy A behavioral therapeutic technique that exposes a client to anxiety-provoking stimuli, through his or her own imagination, in an attempt to extinguish the anxiety associated with the stimuli.

Independent construals of self Conceptualization of the self as an individual whose behavior is organized primarily by reference to one's own thoughts, feelings, and actions, rather than by reference to the thoughts, feelings, and actions of others.

Instrumental aggression Cognition-based and goal-directed aggression carried out with premeditated thought, to achieve specific aims.

Interneurons Brain neurons that relay messages from sensory neurons to other interneurons or to motor neurons.

Ion channels The portions of neurons' cell membranes that selectively permit certain ions to flow in and out.

J

James-Lange theory of emotion A peripheral-feedback theory of emotion stating that an eliciting stimulus triggers a behavioral response that sends different sensory and motor feedback to the brain and creates the feeling of a specific emotion.

K

Ketone. An organic compound containing a carbonyl group $=C=O$ bonded to two hydrocarbon groups, made by oxidizing secondary alcohols. The simplest such compound is acetone.

L

Labile. Liable to change; easily altered. Of or characterized by emotions that are easily aroused or freely expressed, and that tend to alter quickly and spontaneously; emotionally unstable.

Learned helplessness A general pattern of nonresponding in the presence of noxious stimuli that often follows after an organism has previously experienced noncontingent, inescapable aversive stimuli.

Ligand. A molecule that binds to another (usually larger) molecule.

Limbic. The limbic system is a set of brain structures located on both sides of the thalamus, immediately beneath the cerebrum. It has also been referred to as the paleomammalian cortex. It is not a separate system but a collection of structures from the telencephalon, diencephalon, and mesencephalon. The amygdala is the emotion center of the brain, while the hippocampus plays an essential role in the formation of new memories about past experiences.

Limbic system The region of the brain that regulates emotional behavior, basic motivational urges, and memory, as well as major physiological functions.

Lipid hormone. Most lipid hormones are steroid hormones, which are usually ketones or alcohols and are insoluble in water. Steroid hormones (ending in '-ol' or '-one') include estradiol, testosterone, aldosterone, and cortisol. Amino acid–based hormones (amines and peptide or protein hormones) are water-soluble and act on the surface of target cells via second messengers; steroid hormones, being lipid-soluble, move through the plasma membranes of target cells (both cytoplasmic and nuclear) to act within their nuclei.

M

Magnetic resonance imaging (*MRI*). A test that uses powerful magnets, radio waves, and a computer to make detailed pictures inside your body. ... Unlike X-rays and CT scans, an *MRI* doesn't use radiation.. (*MRI*) A test that uses powerful magnets, radio waves, and a computer to make detailed pictures inside your body. Unlike X-rays and CT scans, an *MRI* doesn't use radiation. See also CAT Scan and **Electroencephalogram (EEG).**

Major depressive disorder A mood disorder characterized by intense feelings of depression over an extended time, without the manic high phase of bipolar depression.

Manic episode A component of bipolar disorder characterized by periods of extreme elation, unbounded euphoria without sufficient reason, and grandiose thoughts or feelings about personal abilities.

Medulla The region of the brain stem that regulates breathing, waking, and heartbeat.

Memory The mental capacity to encode, store, and retrieve information.

Metabolism. The chemical processes that occur within a living organism in order to maintain life.

Monoamine. A compound having a single amine group in its molecule, especially one that is a neurotransmitter (e.g., serotonin, norepinephrine).

Monoamine oxidase. An enzyme (present in most tissues) that catalyzes the oxidation and inactivation of monoamine neurotransmitters.

Mood. A temporary state of mind or feeling, such as humor or temper

Mood disorder A mood disturbance such as severe depression or depression alternating with mania.

Motivation The process of starting, directing, and maintaining physical and psychological activities; includes mechanisms involved in preferences for one activity over another and the vigor and persistence of responses.

Motor cortex The region of the cerebral cortex that controls the action of the body's voluntary muscles.

Motor neurons The neurons that carry messages away from the central nervous system toward the muscles and glands.

N

Nature-nurture controversy The debate concerning the relative importance of heredity (nature) and learning or experience (nurture) in determining development and behavior.

Negative reinforcement A behavior is followed by the removal of an aversive stimulus, increasing the probability of that behavior.

Neurogenesis. The growth and development of nervous tissue. In psychology, neurogenesis refers to the process by which neurons or nerve cells are generated in the brain. Neurogenesis is most active during prenatal development, when a baby's brain is being formed. Although it continues through adulthood, new neurons are generated at a much slower pace than during prenatal development.

Neuromodulation. The process by which nervous activity is regulated by way of controlling the physiological levels of several classes of neurotransmitters. Neuromodulators are a subset of neurotransmitter. Unlike neurotransmitters, the release of neuromodulators occurs in a diffuse manner ("volume transmission").

Neuromuscular junction. Is the site of communication between motor nerve axons and muscle fibers. It is composed of four specialized cell types: motor neurons,

Schwann cells, muscle fibers and the recently discovered kranocytes.

Neuron. A specialized cell transmitting nerve impulses; a nerve cell. It receives signals via chemicals called neurotransmitters. It then transmits the signals, electrically. A **neuron** consists of a cell body or soma, dendrites, and a single axon.

Neurotic disorders Mental disorders in which a person does not have signs of brain abnormalities and does not display grossly irrational thinking or violate basic norms but does experience subjective distress; a category dropped from DSM-III.

Neurotransmitter. a chemical substance that is released at the end of a nerve fiber by the arrival of a nerve impulse and, by diffusing across the synapse or junction, causes the transfer of the impulse to another nerve fiber, a muscle fiber, or some other structure.

Neurotrophins. *Neurotrophins* are a family of proteins that induce the survival, development, and function of neurons. They belong to a class of growth factors, secreted proteins that are capable of signaling particular cells to survive, differentiate, or grow.

Noradrenalin. See Norepinephrine.

Norepinephrine. A hormone released by the adrenal medulla and by the sympathetic nerves and functions as a neurotransmitter. It is also used as a drug to raise blood pressure.

Nutrient. A substance that provides nourishment essential for growth and the maintenance of life.

Nutrition. The process of providing or obtaining the food necessary for health and growth. The branch of science that deals with nutrients and nutrition, particularly in humans.

O

Occipital lobe Rearmost region of the brain; contains primary visual cortex.

Operant conditioning Learning in which the probability of a response is changed by a change in its consequences.

Operant extinction When a behavior no longer produces predictable consequences, its return to the level of occurrence it had before operant conditioning.

Oxidase. An enzyme that promotes the transfer of a hydrogen atom from a particular substrate to an oxygen molecule, forming water or hydrogen peroxide.

Oxide. A binary compound of oxygen with another element or group.

P

Pain The body's response to noxious stimuli that are intense enough to cause, or threaten to cause, tissue damage

Parathyroid glands. Are four tiny glands, located in the neck, that control the body's calcium levels. Each gland is about the size of a grain of rice (weighs approximately 30 milligrams and is 3-4 millimeters in diameter). The parathyroids produce a hormone called parathyroid hormone (PTH).

Peptide. A compound consisting of two or more amino acids linked in a chain, the carboxyl group of each acid being joined to the amino group of the next by a bond of the type -OC-NH-.

Peptide hormone. *Peptide hormones* or protein hormones are hormones whose molecules are *peptides* or proteins, respectively. The latter have longer amino acid chain lengths than the former. These *hormones* have an effect on the endocrine system of animals, including humans. *Peptide hormones* represent a major class of *hormones* made from amino acids by specialized endocrine glands. However, excessive amount of circulating *peptide hormones* often associates with the presence of tumors. Peptide hormones are secreted and function in an endocrine manner to regulate many physiological functions, including growth, appetite and energy metabolism, cardiac function, stress, and reproductive physiology. Many signal via G protein-coupled receptors (GPCRs).

Parietal lobe Region of the brain behind the frontal lobe and above the lateral fissure; contains somatosensory cortex

Perception The processes that organize information in the sensory image and interpret it as having been produced by properties of objects or events in the external, three-dimensional world.

PET scans Brain images produced by a device that obtains detailed pictures of activity in the living brain by recording the radioactivity emitted by cells during different cognitive or behavioral activities.

Pharmacology. The branch of medicine concerned with the uses, effects, and modes of action of drugs.

Pituitary gland. The major endocrine gland. A pea-sized body attached to the base of the brain, the pituitary is important in controlling growth and development and the functioning of the other endocrine glands.

Pituitary gland, Anterior.

Pituitary Gland, Anterior. A major organ of the endocrine system, the anterior pituitary (also called the adenohypophysis or parsanterior), is the glandular, anterior lobe that together with the posterior lobe

(posterior pituitary, or the neurohypophysis) makes up
the pituitary gland (hypophysis).

Pons The region of the brain stem that connects the
spinal cord with the brain and links parts of the brain to one
another.

Posterior. Further back in position; of or nearer the
rear or hind end, especially of the body or a part of it.

Posttraumatic stress disorder (PTSD) An anxiety
disorder characterized by the persistent reexperience of
traumatic events through distressing recollections, dreams,
hallucinations, or dissociative flashbacks; develops in
response to rapes, life-threatening events, severe injuries, and
natural disasters.

Problem solving Thinking that is directed toward
solving specific problems and that moves from an initial state
to a goal state by means of a set of mental operations.

Prolactin. A hormone released from the anterior
pituitary gland that stimulates milk production after childbirth.

Postsynaptic neuron. A neuron to the cell body or
dendrite of which an electrical impulse is transmitted across
a synaptic cleft by the release of a chemical neurotransmitter
from the axon terminal of a presynaptic neuron.

Presynaptic neuron. A **neuron** from the axon
terminal of which an electrical impulse is transmitted across
a synaptic cleft to the cell body or one or more dendrites
of a postsynaptic **neuron** by the release of a chemical
neurotransmitter.

Protein hormone. Small peptide *hormones* include
TRH and vasopressin. Peptides composed of scores or
hundreds of amino acids are referred to as *proteins*. Examples
of *protein hormones* include insulin and growth *hormone*. More

complex *protein hormones* bear carbohydrate side-chains and
are called glycoprotein *hormones.*

Psychiatrist An individual who has obtained an
M.D. degree and also has completed postdoctoral specialty
training in mental and emotional disorders; a psychiatrist
may prescribe medications for the treatment of psychological
disorders.

Psychoanalysis. A system of psychological theory and
therapy that aims to treat mental disorders by investigating the
interaction of conscious and unconscious elements in the mind
and bringing repressed fears and conflicts into the conscious
mind by techniques such as dream interpretation and free
association.

Psychoanalyst An individual who has earned either
a Ph.D. or an M.D. degree and has completed postgraduate
training in the Freudian approach to understanding and
treating mental disorders.

Psychodynamic personality theories Theories
of personality that share the assumption that personality is
shaped by and behavior is motivated by powerful inner forces.

Psychodynamic perspective A psychological model
in which behavior is explained in terms of past experiences
and motivational forces; actions are viewed as stemming from
inherited instincts, biological drives, and attempts to resolve
conflicts between personal needs and social requirements.

Psychologist An individual with a doctoral degree
in psychology from an organized, sequential program in a
regionally accredited university or professional school.

Psychosocial stages Proposed by Erik Erikson,
successive developmental stages that focus on an individual's
orientation toward the self and others; these stages
incorporate both the sexual and social aspects of a person's

development and the social conflicts that arise from the interaction between the individual and the social environment.

Psychotherapy. The treatment of mental disorder by psychological rather than medical means.

Psychotic disorders Severe mental disorders in which a person experiences impairments in reality testing manifested through thought, emotional, or perceptual difficulties; no longer used as a diagnostic category after DSM-III.

R

Reasoning The process of thinking in which conclusions are drawn from a set of facts; thinking directed toward a given goal or objective.

Recall A method of retrieval in which an individual is required to reproduce the information previously presented.

Relaxation response A condition in which muscle tension, cortical activity, heart rate, and blood pressure decrease and breathing slows.

Retrieval cues Internally or externally generated stimuli available to help with the retrieval of a memory.

S

SAD

1 Seasonal Affective Disorder. Depression associated with late autumn and winter and thought to be caused by a lack of light.

2 Social Anxiety Disorder. Also called social phobia, is intense anxiety or fear of being judged, negatively evaluated, or rejected in a social or performance situation. People with social anxiety disorder may worry about acting or appearing visibly anxious (e.g., blushing, stumbling over words), or being viewed as stupid, awkward, or boring.

Self-actualization A concept in personality psychology referring to a person's constant striving to realize his or her potential and to develop inherent talents and capabilities.

Self-awareness The top level of consciousness; cognizance of the autobiographical character of personally experienced events.

Self-concept A person's mental model of his or her abilities and attributes.

Self-efficacy The set of beliefs that one can perform adequately in a particular situation.

Self-esteem A generalized evaluative attitude toward the self that influences both moods and behavior and that exerts a powerful effect on a range of personal and social behaviors.

Serotonin. A compound present in blood platelets and serum that constricts the blood vessels and acts as a neurotransmitter.

Social-learning theory The learning theory that stresses the role of observation and the imitation of behaviors observed in others.

Social phobia A persistent, irrational fear that arises in anticipation of a public situation in which an individual can be observed by others.

Social psychology The branch of psychology that studies the effect of social variables on individual behavior, attitudes, perceptions, and motives; also studies group and intergroup phenomena.

Social role A socially defined pattern of behavior that is expected of a person who is functioning in a given setting or group.

Social support Resources, including material aid, socioemotional support, and informational aid, provided by others to help a person cope with stress.

Socialization The lifelong process whereby an individual's behavioral patterns, values, standards, skills, attitudes, and motives are shaped to conform to those regarded as desirable in a particular society.

Steroid hormone. A *steroid* that acts as a *hormone and* grouped into two classes, *corticosteroids* (typically made in the adrenal cortex, hence cortico-) and sex *steroids* (typically made in the gonads or placenta). They have some of the characteristics of true *steroids* as receptor ligands.

Stress The pattern of specific and nonspecific responses an organism makes to stimulus events that disturb its equilibrium and tax or exceed its ability to cope.

Synaptic cleft. The space between neurons at a nerve synapse across which a nerve impulse is transmitted by a neurotransmitter — called also synaptic gap.

Synaptic transmission The relaying of information from one neuron to another across the synaptic gap.

Synaptic vesicles. A small secretory vesicle that contains a neurotransmitter found inside an axon near the presynaptic membrane, and releases its contents into the synaptic cleft after fusing with the membrane

Synapse. A junction between two nerve cells, consisting of a minute gap across which impulses pass by diffusion of a neurotransmitter. The gap between one neuron and another.

Syndrome. A group of symptoms that consistently occur together or a condition characterized by a set of associated symptoms.

T

Temporal lobe Region of brain found below the lateral fissure; contains auditory cortex.

Testosterone. A steroid hormone that stimulates development of male secondary sexual characteristics, produced mainly in the testes, but also in the ovaries and adrenal cortex.

Thalamus. Either of two masses of gray matter lying between the cerebral hemispheres on either side of the third ventricle, relaying sensory information and acting as a center for pain perception

Thyroid. A large cartilage of the larynx, a projection of which forms the Adam's apple in humans.

Thyroid gland. A large ductless gland in the neck that secretes hormones regulating growth and development through the rate of metabolism.

Thyroliberin. A tripeptide hormone produced by the hypothalamus that stimulates the anterior pituitary gland to release thyrotropin. Also called thyrotropin-releasing hormone.

Thyrotropin-releasing factor (TRP). A hormone secreted by the hypothalamus that stimulates release of thyrotropin.

Thyrotropin-releasing hormone (TRH). A hormone secreted by the hypothalamus that stimulates release of thyrotropin.

Tomography. A technique for displaying a representation of a cross section through a human body or other solid object using X-rays or ultrasound.

V

Vasopressin. A pituitary hormone that acts to promote the retention of water by the kidneys and increase blood pressure

Vesicle. A fluid- or air-filled cavity or sac, in particular

W

Wellness Optimal health, incorporating the ability to function fully and actively over the physical, intellectual, emotional, spiritual, social, and environmental domains of health.

Appendix 2

ZUNG SELF-RATING DEPRESSION SCALE

The Zung Self-Rating Depression Scale, designed by W. W. Zung, assesses the level of depression for patients diagnosed with a depressive disorder.

The Zung Self-Rating Depression Scale is a short self-administered survey to quantify the depressed status of a patient. Twenty items appear on the scale that rates the four common characteristics of depression—the pervasive effect, the physiological equivalents, other disturbances, and psychomotor activities.

Ten of the statements are positively worded and ten negatively worded. Each question is scored on a scale of 1-4 (a little of the time, some of the time, good part of the time, most of the time.

The scores range from 20 to 80. Any score from 20 to 50 is considered within the normal range. A score of 51 or more indicates the individual should see a physician, psychiatrist, psychologist, psychological examiner or licensed clinical social worker.

Appendix 3

CHARACTERISTIC SYMPTOMS OF DEPRESSION

Anger or Rage

Anxiety

Chronic Pain

Crying for no Apparent Reason

Decreased/Increased Appetite

Decreased/Increased Sleep

Decreased/Increased Weight

Fatalism

Feeling Totally Discouraged

Feeling Overwhelmed

Feelings of Helplessness

Feelings of Hopelessness

Feelings of Uselessness

Gastrointestinal Problems

Hostility

Hypochondria

Impaired Thinking

Impaired Decision-making

Impaired Memory or Recall

Impaired Concentration Insomnia

Irritability

Insomnia

Irritability

Labile Mood (mood swings)

Lack of Energy

Listlessness (may seem lazy)

Loneliness even around people

Loss of interest: sexual activity

Loss of muscle tone: standing

Lost Interest in favorite activity

Moodiness

Negativity

Periods of short or rapid breath

Sadness – no apparent reason

Sense of despair

Social isolation

Suicidal Ideas or Thoughts

Withdrawal

World better off without me

Appendix 4

GROCERY SUPPLIES FROM FOOD PANTRY

One Month's Groceries from a local non-profit food pantry

REQUIRED FEE FOR PARTICIPATING: $10 MONTHLY

- 1 box Au Gratin potatoes
- 1 box Julienne potatoes
- 1 box sour cream potatoes
- 1 sandwich size paper bag of white rice
- 4 cans cranberry sauce
- 2 cans pigeon peas
- 1 package (10 count) soft Lime Tortillas
- 4 boxes (10 count) corn Taco Shells
- 1 can green salsa
- 1 can vegetarian vegetable soup
- 1 can vegetarian bean soup
- 1 can organic vegetarian split pea soup
- 2 cans unsweetened apple sauce
- 2 boxes Trix cereal (with Hebrew printed on box)
- 1 box of generic corn flakes cereal
- 1 Red Velvet cake (expired date)
- 4 loose peppermint balls, individually wrapped
- 1 loaf French bread
- 1 dozen whole-wheat dinner rolls

2 boxes Little Debbie snack cakes

1 Onion

1 bar soap

1 roll toilet paper

This box and two grocery bags of food stuff and supplies was the monthly provision at a neighborhood food pantry. The recipient of these foods and supplies were for a poverty level individual suffering with depression and diabetes. The person struggled with proper nutrition to ensure weight loss and control of blood sugars for the diabetes. This individual was unable to purchase additional foods at a local grocery (such as meat for the tacos, canned vegetables or fresh produce.

Appendix 5

LIST OF ANTIDEPRESSANT MEDICATIONS BY CLASS

Depression is a mental health issue that starts most often in early adulthood. It is also more common in women. However, anyone at any age may deal with depression.

Depression affects your brain, so drugs that work in your brain may prove beneficial. Common antidepressants may help ease your symptoms, but there are many other options as well. Each drug used to treat depression works by balancing certain chemicals in your brain called neurotransmitters. These drugs work in slightly different ways to ease your depression symptoms.

Many common drugs fall into the following drug classes:

- selective serotonin reuptake inhibitors (SSRIs)
- serotonin and norepinephrine reuptake inhibitors (SNRIs)
- tricyclic antidepressants (TCAs)
- tetracyclic antidepressant
- dopamine reuptake blocker
- 5-HT1A receptor antagonist
- 5-HT2 receptor antagonists
- 5-HT3 receptor antagonist
- monoamine oxidase inhibitors (MAOIs)
- noradrenergic antagonist

Atypical antidepressants, which don't fall into these drug classes, and natural treatments such as St. John's wort (See note at end) are also available.

Selective serotonin reuptake inhibitors (SSRIs)

SSRIs are the most commonly prescribed class of antidepressants. An imbalance of serotonin may play a role in depression. These drugs fight depression symptoms by decreasing serotonin reuptake in your brain. This effect leaves more serotonin available to work in your brain.

SSRIs include:

- sertraline (Zoloft)
- fluoxetine (Prozac, Sarafem)
- citalopram (Celexa)
- escitalopram (Lexapro)
- paroxetine (Paxil, Pexeva, Brisdelle)
- fluvoxamine (Luvox)

Common side effects of SSRIs include:

- nausea
- trouble sleeping
- nervousness
- tremors
- sexual problems

Serotonin and norepinephrine reuptake inhibitors (SNRIs)

SNRIs help improve serotonin and norepinephrine levels in your brain. This may reduce depression symptoms.

SNRIs include:

- desvenlafaxine (Pristiq, Khedezla)
- duloxetine (Cymbalta)
- levomilnacipran (Fetzima)
- venlafaxine (Effexor XR)

In addition to treating depression, duloxetine may also relieve pain. This is important because chronic pain can lead to depression or make it worse. In some cases, people with depression become more aware of aches and pains. A drug that treats both depression and pain, such as duloxetine, can be helpful to these people.

Common side effects of SNRIs include:

- nausea
- drowsiness
- fatigue
- constipation
- dry mouth

Tricyclic antidepressants (TCAs)

TCAs are often prescribed when SSRIs or other antidepressants don't work. It isn't fully understood how these drugs work to treat depression.

TCAs include:

- amitriptyline
- amoxapine
- clomipramine (Anafranil)
- desipramine (Norpramin)
- doxepin

- <u>imipramine</u> (Tofranil)
- <u>nortriptyline</u> (Pamelor)
- <u>protriptyline</u>
- trimipramine (<u>Surmontil</u>)

Common side effects of TCAs can include:

- constipation
- dry mouth
- fatigue
- The more serious side effects of these drugs include:
- low blood pressure
- irregular heart rate
- seizures

Tetracyclic antidepressant

<u>Maprotiline</u> is used to treat depression and anxiety. It also works by balancing neurotransmitters to ease symptoms of depression.

- <u>Maprotiline</u>

Common side effects of this drug include:

- drowsiness
- weakness
- lightheadedness
- headache
- blurry vision
- dry mouth

Dopamine reuptake blocker

Bupropion (Wellbutrin, Forfivo, Aplenzin) is a mild dopamine and norepinephrine reuptake blocker. It's used for depression and seasonal affective disorder. It's also used in smoking cessation.

- Bupropion
- Wellbutrin
- Forfivo
- Aplenzin

Common side effects include:

- nausea
- vomiting
- constipation
- dizziness
- blurry vision

5-HT1A receptor antagonist

The drug in this class that's used to treat depression is called vilazodone(Viibryd). It works by balancing serotonin levels and other neurotransmitters. This drug is rarely used as a first-line treatment for depression. That means it's usually only prescribed when other medications didn't work for you or caused bothersome side effects.

Side effects can include:

- nausea
- vomiting
- trouble sleeping

5-HT2 receptor antagonists

Two 5-HT2 receptor antagonists, nefazodone and trazodone (Oleptro), are used to treat depression. These are older drugs. They alter chemicals in your brain to help depression.

*   nefazodone
*   trazodone

Common side effects include:

*   drowsiness
*   dizziness
*   dry mouth

5-HT3 receptor antagonist

The 5-HT3 receptor antagonist vortioxetine (Brintellix) treats depression by affecting the activity of brain chemicals.

*   Brintellix

Common side effects include:

*   sexual problems
*   nausea

Monoamine oxidase inhibitors (MAOIs)

MAOIs are older drugs that treat depression. They work by stopping the breakdown of norepinephrine, dopamine, and serotonin. They're more difficult for people to take than most other antidepressants because they interact with prescription drugs, nonprescription drugs, and some foods. They also can't be combined with stimulants or other antidepressants.

MAOIs include:

*   isocarboxazid (Marplan)
*   phenelzine (Nardil)

- selegiline (Emsam), which comes as a transdermal patch
- tranylcypromine (Parnate)

MAOIs also have many side effects. These can include:

- nausea
- dizziness
- drowsiness
- trouble sleeping
- restlessness

Noradrenergic antagonist

Mirtazapine (Remeron) is used primarily for depression. It alters certain chemicals in your brain to ease depression symptoms.

- Mirtazapine

Common side effects include:

- drowsiness
- dizziness
- weight gain

Atypical medications

Other depression drugs do not fall into the typical classes. These are called atypical antidepressants. Depending on your condition, your doctor may prescribe one of these alternatives instead.

For example, olanzapine/fluoxetine (Symbyax) is an atypical antidepressant. It is used to treat bipolar disorder and major depression that does not respond to other drugs.

- olanzapine/fluoxetine

Natural treatments

You may be interested in natural options to treat your depression. Some people use these treatments instead of drugs, and some use them as an add-on treatment to their antidepressant medication.

A WORD OF CAUTION ABOUT ST. JOHN'S WORT:

St. John's wort is an herb that some people have tried for depression. According to the National Center of Complementary and Integrative Health, the herb may have mild positive effects, or it may not work any better than placebo. *This herb also causes many drug interactions that can be serious*. It does not work with certain medications.

St. John's wort interacts with:

- antiseizure drugs
- birth control pills
- Warfarin (Coumadin)
- prescription antidepressants

Living With A Dead Battery

Depression:

A Primer for Family and Professionals

About The Author

Donald B. Smith, MSSW, DPhil, LCSW (Ret.)

Board Certified Diplomate in Clinical Social Work

Dr. Smith has spent 56 years as a social worker and teacher. His background in social work includes the fields of inpatient and outpatient mental health, geriatrics, adolescent reeducation and counseling, hospice, and adoption. His first social work job was as a group worker and recreation leader for children and adolescents at a United Methodist Church urban community center in an inner city neighborhood in Chattanooga, Tennessee USA. His last social work job was as a child protection social worker in adoptions division for the County of Los Angeles (CA) Department of Children and Family Services. In this position he had an active caseload of 158 children.

Donald B. Smith was the first social worker in the Tennessee Adolescent Reeducation Center, the nation's 2nd adolescent inpatient treatment facility, where he supervised liaison teacher counselors who worked with schools and families of children with educational and substance abuse issues. Dr. Smith also pioneered geriatric mental health services in both outpatient and inpatient facilities and was the first Board Certified Clinical Social Worker in the United States in the field of geriatrics.

In 1965 Dr. Smith organized the first integrated Boy Scout Troop in the Southern United States that comprised the 11 deep-south states of the "old Confederacy." He was an early proponent of equal rights for women. A former governor of the State of Tennessee has recognized Dr. Smith as an "Outstanding Tennessean" for his work. He also was awarded the Citizenship Award by the John Sevier Chapter of the Sons of the American Revolution.

Serving as a Scoutmaster and Sea Scout Skipper for a total of 35 years, Dr. Smith was fortunate to have 22 Eagle Scouts and 3 Quartermaster Scouts earn their program's highest awards. For most of those years, he had to fund these inner city programs out of his own pocket in order to pay for membership fees, charter fees, program fees, supplies, and equipment. He also provided a boat for the Sea Scout Ship.

Dr. Smith paid the way for 6 inner city Scouts to attend Boy Scout National Jamborees. While serving in the military in San Antonio Texas, he kept his Scout troop registered during this time and provided leadership to his boy leaders via mail. Dr. Smith took his leave time from the Army to drive back to Chattanooga Tennessee to take his inner city Boy Scout Troop to Summer Camp. It was at these summer camps where his Scouts made their advancement in ranks and earned merit badges. His Scout Troop was the first integrated troop to attend a formerly all-white week at the camp.

Dr. Smith has been a member of the Lion's Club, the American Legion, the United States Coast Guard Auxiliary, the United Methodist Church, and the National Association of Social Workers. He is a past president

DEPRESSION: A PRIMER FOR FAMILY & PROFESSIONALS   219

of the Tennessee Association of Health Care Social
Workers.

Dr. Smith has held social work licenses in the
states of Alabama, Georgia, and Tennessee. He is a
Board Certified Diplomate in Clinical Social Work and
the Academy of Clinical Social Workers. He has held
memberships in the Council on Social Work Education,
American Geriatric Society, the Gerontological Society
of America, the Child Welfare League, and the National
Federation of Settlement Houses and Neighborhood
Centers.

The founding Executive Director for the United
Methodist Inner City Ministry for Chattanooga District of
Holston Conference, Dr. Smith also served as a local
church coordinator for a hospitality network for homeless
families. He was a volunteer director of the Hands
Across the River Parish, an urban parish of 4 north
shore and downtown United Methodist Churches in the
Chattanooga District, Holston Conference.

Dr. Smith has a double Master of Science in Social
Work degree from the University of Tennessee, in Social
Work Administration and in Community Organization.
His clinical training was in the Department of
Neuropsychiatry, US Army Medical Field Service School,
Brooke Army Medical Center in San Antonio Texas,
where he also received training for classroom instructors.
His doctorate is in the Sociological Integration of Religion
and Society from Omega (née Oxford) Graduate School.

www.ingramcontent.com/pod-product-compliance
Lightning Source LLC
Chambersburg PA
CBHW050649270326
41927CB00012B/2942